Dewey Tull Lawson

PRIMER OF ALLERGY

PRIMER OF ALLERGY

A GUIDEBOOK FOR THOSE WHO MUST FIND THEIR WAY THROUGH THE MAZES OF THIS STRANGE AND TANTALIZING STATE

BY

WARREN T. VAUGHAN, M.S., M.D.
Richmond, Virginia

With Illustrations by John P. Tillery

FOURTH EDITION

REVISED BY

J. HARVEY BLACK, M.D.
Dallas, Texas

ST. LOUIS
THE C. V. MOSBY COMPANY
1954

Printed in the
United States of America

Press of
The C. V. Mosby Company
St. Louis

TO MY ASSOCIATE AND FRIEND

W. RANDOLPH GRAHAM, M.D.

PREFACE TO FOURTH EDITION

The demand for a fourth edition of this little book is the very best evidence of the worth of the method of presentation which Doctor Vaughan devised. Evidently it meets the needs of the reader so we have made no effort to change it. We have added a chapter on the drugs commonly used in allergic conditions and we have tried to make it an integral part of the "military picture" used throughout the book.

The changes in this edition are much more extensive than in the last. Some of the new material is necessitated by the accumulation of new knowledge, and some changes have been made in an effort to meet more completely the needs of the reader. We have tried to provide the answers to the many questions which arise in the minds of those who suffer from allergic conditions.

If the frequent reference to foods as the cause of allergy leaves the impression that foods are considered the most frequent and the most important allergens, let us correct that impression. We do believe that foods are frequent causes of allergic reactions but the reason for the seeming emphasis on them is only that they serve as useful and easily understood examples and lend themselves well to the method of discussion. Certainly, the inhalants are of paramount importance in a large share of the allergic conditions we see.

It has been our experience that the better informed the patient is, the better the result we get in his treatment. So we hope this book will serve a useful purpose in telling the patient about his illness, what can be done about it, and how intelligent cooperation makes good results possible. If it fulfills this purpose we shall be pleased.

HARVEY BLACK

PREFACE TO THIRD EDITION

Like the other publications of Dr. Vaughan, the *Primer* proved to be a very popular book. Written with the authority derived from his great knowledge and wide experience, it became a source book for the patient suffering from allergy and the general practitioner with a limited experience in this field; even the specialists often found it helpful.

There are many competent physicians but few who can frame their teaching in such fashion that it is both interesting and intelligible to those not versed in medical terminology. Dr. Vaughan had this facility, as demonstrated by this volume, and this accounted, in large degree, for the popularity of the *Primer*.

Dr. Vaughan died before the time came to bring this book up to date and the pleasant task of revising it has been given to me. In attempting it I have felt that it was quite important to leave unchanged the form of presentation. I could not think of any way to improve it. I have made what changes were required by the advances in knowledge and have added here and there the information which has been accumulating since the printing of the last edition. It is otherwise the same book, brought up to date much as I believe Dr. Vaughan would have had it if he had lived to do it himself.

HARVEY BLACK

Dallas, Texas

PREFACE TO FIRST EDITION

When, in 1930, the author undertook the writing of his first book on allergy, the subject was sufficiently in its infancy that he could successfully incorporate in a single volume pertinent information of interest to physician and patient alike. This was still possible although distinctly more difficult in 1934 when the second edition of *Allergy and Applied Immunology* made its appearance. When a third edition was called for, it was realized that one volume would suffice only by sacrificing too much of the story as it should be prepared for physicians or by forcing upon the lay reader a great mass of technical information in which he is not especially interested.

The only satisfactory solution appeared to be the preparation of two separate volumes, one addressed to the doctor and the other to the patient. While the former, *Practice of Allergy,* has grown to a volume of well over a thousand large, closely typed pages, the latter has been reduced to what the author hopes will be adjudged a reasonably good bedtime story.

The volume is distinctly utilitarian since it was created to fulfill a need, which the writer has experienced, for a small A-B-C of the subject from which his patients may attain sufficient insight into their problem to be able to cooperate intelligently in the effort to bring them relief from their vexing symptoms. Since other physicians treating the same maladies have often mentioned the need for a book of this type, it has been so arranged that it may be similarly used by others, even though their approach to the subject and their selection of therapeutic measures may be at variance with those of the writer. The author hopes that these others may find that it will be of service to them. If in addition it enables the individual who experiences allergic symptoms to gain a more rational insight, and to adjust himself with greater success to those environmental factors which contribute to his discomfort, then the writer will feel that the task was worth the effort.

Since this is intended primarily as a companion piece to the larger volume, bibliographic references and acknowledgments of the investigations of others, all of which appear therein, have, for simplification, been omitted. The writer's deep appreciation of their very important contributions to the study of allergy is, however, undiminished.

These investigators will eventually solve the riddle of allergy. Until then relief for its victims must be achieved, in so far as possible, according to the principles outlined in this book.

The author deeply appreciates the permission granted him by H. T. Webster and the *New York Herald Tribune* to include Mr. Webster's cartoons. The illustration on page 39 was prepared by my niece, Dr. Elizabeth Vaughan; those heading chapters and the final one were drawn by Mr. John P. Tillery.

W. T. V.

Richmond, Virginia.

CONTENTS

CHAPTER IX

CHAPTER X

CHAPTER XI

CHAPTER XII

ILLUSTRATIONS

PRIMER OF ALLERGY

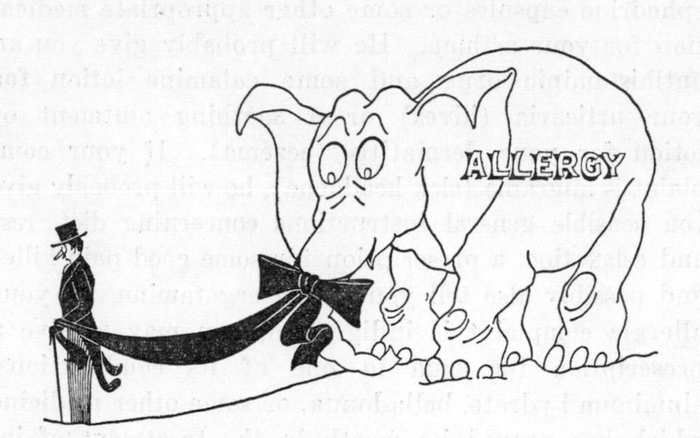

Man's White Elephant

I

LEARN TO LIVE WITH YOUR ALLERGY

Are you a victim of allergy? If so, you have plenty of company. About sixteen million other persons living in the United States are in the same predicament. And sick enough to require a doctor's aid.

What happens when you, who are allergic, seek help from the doctor? As a rule you will first go either to your family physician or to a diagnostician. He will tell you what is the matter with you and give you medicine to relieve the immediate symptoms. It may be nose drops or an "antihistaminic" drug for your hay fever or an injection of epinephrine or some

---

Reprinted by permission of *Life and Health.*

ephedrine capsules or some other appropriate medication for your asthma. He will probably give you an antihistaminic drug and some calamine lotion for your urticaria (hives) or a soothing ointment or lotion for your dermatitis (eczema). If your complaint is migraine (sick headache), he will probably give you sensible general instructions concerning diet, rest and relaxation, a prescription for some good pain killer and possibly also tell you to try ergotamine. If your allergic complaint is indigestion, you may receive a prescription for soda in one of its combinations, aluminum hydrate, belladonna, or some other medicine which has proved its worth in the treatment of indigestion. He may tell you to avoid roughage, fibrous material in the diet, and if he is on his toes, he may tell you to avoid certain foods which past experience has taught him may affect persons unfavorably. The list will include such delicacies as shellfish, onions, chocolate, cabbage, melons, cucumber, tomatoes, strawberries, spices, and the like.

These methods are appropriate for relieving symptoms and you will soon be feeling better. But, if you are allergic, improvement will be only temporary. You will continue with the treatment, but when you find that it is only while doing so that you are even halfway comfortable, you will become discouraged.

By now you have discussed your symptoms with the doctor many times and he is commencing to get as tired of them as you are. He has tried out many variations of the schedule which he originally outlined for you. Some have failed. Most have helped but improvement has always been temporary and dependent upon continued use of the medicine.

At about this stage of the game you go to a bridge party. There, you describe your symptoms and tell of your discouragement. One friend suddenly becomes interested. "Why," she announces, "you are allergic!" This word is not altogether new to you. You have seen it in the newspapers and in cartoons. You have probably heard it in a movie or two. You have gathered the impression that "to be allergic" implies that you do not tolerate something or someone—that although most people get along very nicely on exposure to or contact with some particular substance, the person who is allergic to it does not. For practical purposes this is as good a definition as any. Your friend tells you of the many tests that may be done to discover what substance may be causing your difficulties. It may be a food: wheat, egg, milk, chocolate, tomatoes, melons, shellfish. It may be something that you are breathing: house dust, feather dust, cosmetics, emanations from animals, dogs, cat, horses. It may be pollens. Possibly it is a supposedly harmless drug such as aspirin or some laxative that you are taking. It may be something which, although harmless to the skins of most people, irritates yours. This might be some article of clothing, your jewelry, your nail polish, or even the ointments that you are using to relieve your dermatitis.

By now all the ladies in the room are interested in your case. Tradition has it that in former times when two or more ladies were gathered together they adored talking about their operations. Today they adore talking about their allergies. It is truly a subject for general conversation. With ten persons the probability is that at least one has had to see the doctor about it. Furthermore, investigators have found evidence that about one-half the population has some mild allergic symptom at some time. One doctor has reported that 45 per cent of the families which he surveyed had at least one case. So, if the ladies at the bridge party have not had it themselves, they are likely to know someone who has.

It is a delightful subject for general conversation. First, you can talk about yourself. Second, you can be mysterious, saying, "I knew someone who—." Third, some of the experiences of allergic patients are extremely interesting; some are fantastic. Some are true while others have been exaggerated in the telling. Among the true ones we might mention the man who had a hay fever when smoking Old Gold cigarettes but not after Pall Malls; the woman who was allergic to her bedroom furniture, sensitized to the lacquer covering it; the man who had eczema on an unmentionable part of his anatomy because he was allergic to the paint on his toilet seat; the breast-fed infant who developed eczema whenever his mother ate eggs; the child sensitized to cottonseed who had allergy when he drank cow's milk if the cow had been fed cottonseed meal.

You leave the party wondering why your doctor did not know all about this. Bright and early the next morning you are in his office with fire in your eye. He soon reassures you. Some of his patients have been relieved with the treatment which he has given you. He may tell you of some other equally interesting anecdotes in his own experience. He has not sent you to an allergist because allergic studies are expensive. At that, you rapidly calculate how much money you have spent on drugs and wonder whether, all told, it could be more expensive.

At this point the doctor will do either of two things. If he has become allergic to your complaint, he will refer you to an allergist, happy to have someone share responsibility. If not, he will tell you that he can do a few allergy tests which may solve your problem. If you are allergic to just a few common allergens, this is all that will be necessary. If your allergy is complicated you may still have to consult an allergist. Fifty per

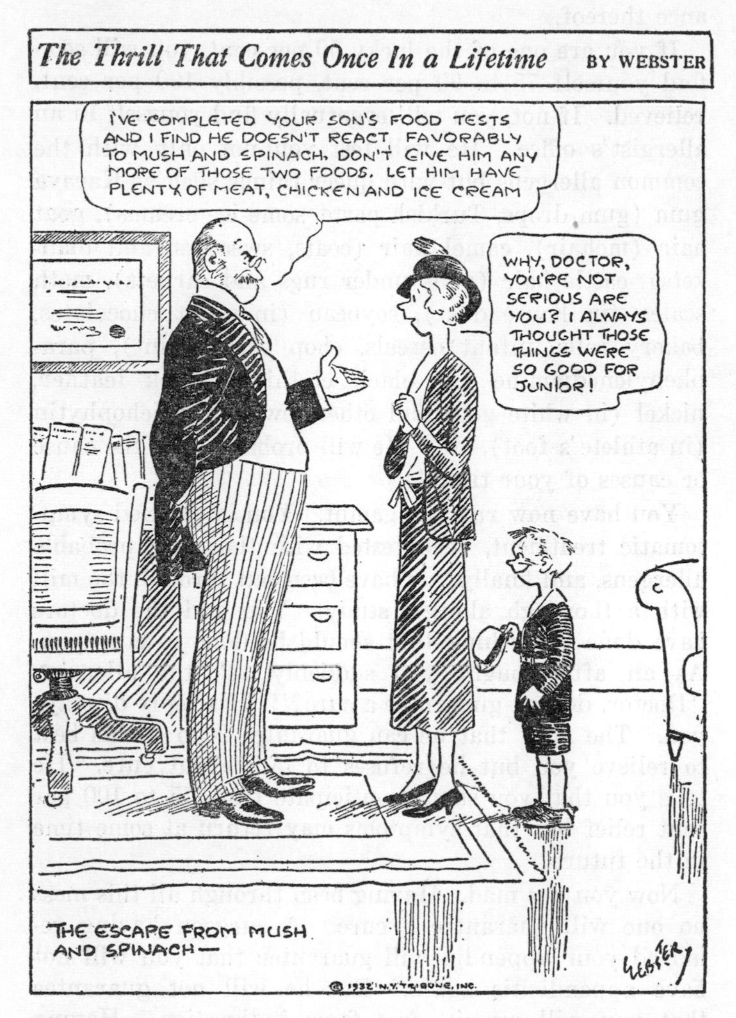

The Thrill That Comes Once In a Lifetime
BY WEBSTER
I'VE COMPLETED YOUR SON'S FOOD TESTS AND I FIND HE DOESN'T REACT FAVORABLY TO MUSH AND SPINACH. DON'T GIVE HIM ANY MORE OF THOSE TWO FOODS. LET HIM HAVE PLENTY OF MEAT, CHICKEN AND ICE CREAM
WHY, DOCTOR, YOU'RE NOT SERIOUS ARE YOU? I ALWAYS THOUGHT THOSE THINGS WERE SO GOOD FOR JUNIOR!
THE ESCAPE FROM MUSH AND SPINACH—
WEBSTER
© 1932 N.Y. TRIBUNE, INC.

(Published by permission of *New York Herald Tribune.*)

cent of allergics are sensitized only to the common offenders and can be reasonably well relieved by avoidance thereof.

If you are one of the lucky 50 per cent, you will soon find yourself 75 to 90 per cent, possibly 100 per cent, relieved. If not, you will eventually find yourself in an allergist's office. He will test you not only with the common allergens but with queer things such as Karaya gum (gum drops, Turkish paste, some ice creams), goat hair (mohair), camel hair (coats, sweaters, and blankets), cattle hair (pads under rugs and carpets), moth scales (in house dust), soybean (in sweet chocolates, bakery rolls, infant cereals, chop suey, paint), paraphenylenediamine (in black clothing, black leather, nickel (in white gold and other jewelry), trichophytin (in athlete's foot), etc. He will probably find the cause or causes of your trouble.

You have now run the gamut. You have tried symptomatic treatment, been tested with the more probable allergens, and finally you have been put through the mill with a thorough allergic study. You and the doctors have done everything that should be done to cure you. As an afterthought you suddenly ask the allergist, "Doctor, do you guarantee a cure?" His reply dismays you. The most that he can guarantee is to do his best to relieve you but he refuses to talk about cure. He tells you that you should anticipate from 75 to 100 per cent relief but that symptoms may return at some time in the future.

Now you *are* mad. Having been through all this mess no one will guarantee a cure. A surgeon having removed your appendix will guarantee that you will not have appendicitis again. But he will not guarantee that you will remain free from indigestion. Having removed a stomach ulcer he cannot assure you that another ulcer will not form under certain circumstances.

Having removed your gall bladder, he cannot guarantee that you will not have trouble from infection of the bile passages. The internist who has helped you through severe bronchitis and pneumonia cannot assure you that you will never have another attack.

But there are very particular reasons why your allergy may return. Let us analyze them.

First, allergy seems to be an hereditary disease. The tendency to become sensitized or allergic to things is inherited. The doctor might find every single thing that you are allergic to now and if you can avoid them satisfactorily, you will get 100 per cent relief. Even if you cannot avoid them completely, he can build up your resistance to them by means of injections and you may still get 100 per cent relief. But this will not destroy the inherited tendency to become sensitized to things. So, you might become allergic to new substances at some time in the future. This tendency is not such that one picks up new allergies every few days, as some people seem to think, but over a period of months there may be changes. If one stops eating a food to which he is sensitive, after a period of time, usually several months or a year or more, he may lose this sensitivity. And, over a period of months, he may develop a new one. We once had the opportunity of watching a woman become sensitive to one thing after another and the shortest time required, even though the exposure was marked, was nine months.

The influence of an hereditary factor could be bred out if marriage could be controlled but people are not going to be deterred from marrying because the intended spouse may be allergic. Allergy is not considered an important obstacle to matrimony.

Another reason why symptoms may persist is the difficulty of avoiding offending allergens. I said just now that if one cannot completely avoid an allergen, the doctor can increase one's resistance by desensitizing injections. This will usually protect against moderate exposure to the allergen but is not guaranteed against unusually heavy exposure. If one is sensitized to the hair of one's favorite puppy dog, injections will probably protect against the amount of exposure that one would have visiting in a house where dogs had been but would probably not protect against using your dog as a cheek warmer. Hay fever injections will give you much relief during the pollen season but on those few days when the pollen concentration in the air is unusually high you may still have symptoms.

A third possible reason for continuance of symptoms is what we call multiple sensitization. It is rather unusual for a person to be allergic just to one thing. One is usually sensitized to several environmental factors or foods. Here we must be reasonable. We must explain that if you will avoid most of the positive foods you will probably feel much better, although you will continue to have some trouble. Few patients are reasonable in this respect. They want complete relief. If they do not get it, they blame the doctor, failing to realize that it was not the doctor who made them allergic in the first place.

A fourth reason for failure is that there is always a small percentage of people in whom, try as he may, the physician fails to secure adequate relief. It may be due to an error in diagnosis or some mistake in treatment. It may be due to some factor about which we yet know nothing. Practically no disease can be cured in every instance and in the care of the allergic patients we occasionally find one to whom we can give no help and we have no explanation for the failure.

The fifth and one of the most important causes for failure of satisfactory relief is lack of understanding and cooperation on the part of the patient. You, the patient, go to the doctor subconsciously expecting him to wave a wand and pronounce you well. If he gives you desensitizing injections, you feel sure that this will turn the trick and that you can go ahead as in the past doing whatever you wish, with impunity. It does not work that way.

In allergy more than in any other type of illness one must learn to adjust oneself to those deleterious environmental influences (foods, inhalants, medicines, contact substances, even emotional problems) toward which one has developed an idiosyncrasy. The allergic tendency being inherited, one must learn to live with one's allergy with a minimum of resulting discomfort. Among other things this depends upon close attention to details in carrying out the doctor's instructions and in abiding by them. The doctor can tell you what you should do but you will not get best results unless you actually do it. A lady living in a distant town was instructed how to rid her room of dust, feathers, and kapok. For several months she wrote that she was no better. Then she gleefully announced that she had cured herself. In rearranging her furniture she had removed a studio couch from her bedroom. This was stuffed with kapok. Had she carried out the original instructions she would have saved herself several months of asthma.

A lion tamer gets into no difficulty as long as he remembers that there is something dangerous in his immediate environment, and exercises appropriate precautions to protect himself. The man with allergy should do likewise. Fortunately the situation is not quite as bad since prolonged avoidance usually seems to result in loss of sensitization and treatment over a sufficiently long period may bring about permanent relief. Then, too, we see persons occasionally who have a "spontaneous cure" or, as it is usually expressed, they "outgrow" their allergy. While not so common an event as is usually believed, it does sometimes occur. In this sense there is hope of actual cure but until the doctor has announced that such exposures will be safe, he who wishes maximum comfort must adjust himself to his environment or vice versa. He must learn to live with his allergy.

II

ABRACADABRA

Abracadabra is a cabalistic word, a word-charm used by ancient peoples to help ward off disease. Although it appears to be but meaningless jargon, when separated into its component parts it becomes a fancy way of saying A, B, C, D. Somehow, when spoken quickly, it brings to mind pictures of Hindu fakirs waving wands, doing hocus pocus, and bringing rabbits out of hats. Well, we have no rabbits to produce and allergy certainly cannot be treated by the waving of a wand. Herein, you will find the A-B-C of allergy, the perusal of which, it is hoped, will help you to ward off the symptoms of this curious malady.

There is much that is mysterious in allergy. Why should one person react with symptoms of severe illness, following contact with or exposure to a substance which is perfectly harmless, even beneficial, to the vast majority of human beings? One would think that wild flowers, grasses, and trees were placed upon the earth for us to admire and enjoy. They offer beauty, comfort, or pleasing shade, and we are grateful for them. And yet there are those who cannot get within the vicinity of these without developing fits of coughing and tightness in the chest which increase rapidly in severity until the victim is gasping for breath and thoroughly ill.

There are others who react differently. They sneeze. They sneeze again. Soon there is a regular staccato of sneezing, reminiscent of machine gun barrages during the war. The lining membrane in the nose swells full with fluid, closing off these upper air passages, and soon the fluid leaks through the surfaces, flowing from the nose in great abundance.

A few who eat honey find that soon thereafter something seems to go wrong in their heads and such a pain develops on one side or both that its possessor wonders whether ten thousand imprisoned impish devils are using sledge hammers, trying to break their way out.

Man and his dog have been inseparable companions since before the dawn of earliest history, yet there are those who cannot pet a dog without breaking out with an itching rash, with great red wheals resembling the bites of dozens of bees.

Bread is the staff of life, but some who eat it find that it causes violent commotions inside the abdomen, not relieved until it has been promptly removed by vomiting or, more slowly, with diarrhea.

Clothing has enabled us to live in parts of the earth where it would otherwise be impossible, but some find that certain types of clothing produce a chronic breaking-out of the skin, an eczema of the more irritating variety. A few of us would indeed find peace and freedom from interminable scratching only after joining a nudist colony.

Doctors have perfected medicines, drugs which are indispensable for the treatment and cure of disease. Some there are who, even though the nature of their illness calls loudly for its administration, cannot take a particular drug without developing one of the symptoms just described, asthma, hay fever or allergic rhinitis, sick headache or migraine, urticaria, gastrointestinal allergy, allergic dermatitis, or some other less common and more obscure response, such as disappearance of many of the protective white corpuscles from the blood (agranulocytosis) or of the little platelets whose function it is to cause the blood to clot (thrombocytopenic purpura).

Man has worshipped the sun as the source of life and health since earliest times. We still see evidence of sun worship in the cult of sun tanners, the bathers who at the beach strip to the farthest limits of decency, and in the ultraviolet light machines which doctors use. There are some, however, who cannot tolerate prolonged exposure to the sun's rays without becoming violently ill with a severe skin eruption, quite different from sunburn, or with gastrointestinal upsets or even collapse and unconsciousness. Others react in this curious way upon exposure to cold water. Many "accidental" drownings are attributed to such an abnormal response.

If this be allergy, surely it is a mysterious malady. What happens in an individual to make him react in such a curious and violent way after contact with extraneous substances which are harmless, nay beneficial, to others? Why will one such victim respond to the eating of eggs with an attack of hay fever while another has migraine and a third cramp-colic or colitis? Why don't all respond to the same food with the same symptoms? Why does ragweed cause hay fever in one, asthma in another, and eczema in a third? Why does one asthmatic have trouble from inhaling house dust, another from feather dust, a third from eating cantaloupe and a fourth after the hypodermic injection of a curative horse serum? Why shouldn't the cause of asthma be the same in all?

What may be done about it? How may we determine which of these harmless substances are harmful for the individual and what steps may be taken to render them harmless again? There is much of which we are still ignorant in allergy but in the last third of a century many things have been learned and, fortunately, have been applied in the treatment of this strange disease.

In the pages which follow, the author will attempt to explain the Abracadabra of Allergy in not-too-technical terms. Some of its phases, such as the technical theories of the biochemical alterations in the allergic response, are too involved and indeed are not altogether understood by experts who have devoted a lifetime to their study. These will therefore be touched on only briefly, particularly so since this is intended primarily as a guide book for the patient seeking quickest relief from his illness, and their importance is therefore secondary to that of "what to do about it."

Antiquity

Although you probably never heard the term before a few years ago, allergy is not a new disease. Today it is so widely recognized, not only by the medical profession but by the public at large, that it has become a household word. Ogden Nash has written poems concerning it, Webster and other famous cartoonists have used it as a source of fun, and even Ginger Rogers of movie fame has carried the word to millions of ears, across the meshes of the silver screen. Indeed, at tea parties, if there are tea parties any more, and certainly at bridge parties, milady no longer compares her experiences at her last operation with those of her neighbor, but much prefers to discuss the mysteries of her allergic manifestations.

Although not a new disease, allergy as a word was unknown prior to 1905 when a famous Viennese physician coined it to describe this curiously altered capacity to react to those things with which we come into contact. The word, translated from the Greek, literally means "altered energy" or "altered reactivity." Although the name first appeared within our century, and only since then have we reached sufficient understanding of the malady to be able to do something about it, the disease itself has existed since earliest times. Before then we called it idiosyncrasy. Idiosyncrasy, literally translated, means very much the same thing: "a reaction peculiar to the individual."

So we find an old friend so dressed up in new togs as to be scarcely recognizable. We find him much more interesting. He is much less mysterious. Formerly we just acknowledged an old acquaintance named Mr. Idiosyncrasy, and passed him by. Now we are interested. We study him, analyze him, take him apart and put him together again as it were, find his weak points, and can combat him with the knowledge thus attained. Some of you can remember when people had "catarrh." They still do but now we call it allergic rhinitis, nasal allergy, or perennial hay fever. The condition is the same—the name has been changed to conform to new knowledge of it.

Hippocrates, the earliest writer on medicine, who lived 400 years before Christ, described idiosyncrasy to cheese, which today we would recognize as allergy. Lucretius, one hundred years before Christ, originated the expression so often quoted today, to the effect that one man's meat is another's poison. However, Lucretius was a better allergist than those who have translated his words, since he did not write precisely this. He wrote that "what is food for some *may* be an intense poison for others," implying thereby that not all other persons will *necessarily* find it harmful.

Students of the history of medicine find similar passages in the writings of nearly all centuries since Hippocrates, clearly indicating that allergy is not a new disease.

We are frequently asked if allergies are not much more frequent than they used to be and the answer must be that no one knows. We can be sure that allergy to drugs is much more frequent than formerly due to the enormous number of new, synthetic drugs. But there is no reliable evidence that hay fever and asthma are more common than they were years ago. Probably the reason for this seeming increase is the fact that we now have a great deal of interest in them, talk a lot about them, and do something for them. They used to be accepted as a dispensation of Providence about which nothing could be done so they were tolerated in relative silence. An instructor in medical school once remarked that you never know how many wooden legs there are until you lose your own leg. You never realize how common asthma may be until you or a member of your family suffers from it.

New Words

Are you in the radio business? If so, you have found it necessary to employ words which you never used before, such as antenna, heterodyne, neutrodyne, radiobroadcast and television. Possibly you are in the automobile business. Before motor cars were built there was no need for words such as carburetor, clutch, chassis, differential, garage. New machines and mechanisms, new methods of government and new developments in scientific research require the coining of new terms to describe articles or phenomena which were previously unknown, so that they may be differentiated from others. In science it is customary to go back to the Greek or Latin roots to coin new words. Each separate part of the new word actually signifies something in Greek or Latin and this original significance is still retained in the new word. Velocipede might be literally translated as "a fast foot." An automobile is something which moves itself.

Another method in naming new things is to adopt a word already in existence but which has previously been used with different connotation, but with a traceable resemblance. The wireless antenna reminds one of the antennae on the head of a butterfly. The clutch is something which grabs, as all who have driven Model T Fords will agree.

When our old friend Idiosyncrasy became of scientific interest and was taken apart, the parts had to be named. This just makes it easier to talk about them. If I had to describe a carburetor as that-little-round-brass-thing-under-the-hood-into - which - gasoline - flows -

from -a-copper-tube-and-air-enters - from-a - large - vent-where-both-are-mixed-up-together-and-discharged - as - a-vapor-into-the-cylinders, I would have very little time left to say what I actually started out to say.

There are not many terms in allergy with which you must become acquainted to be able readily to understand this book, so we might as well get at them without further ado.

Idiosyncrasy (Greek *idios,* one's own, + *synkrasis,* a mixing together). Chemically, a mixing together is a reaction. One's own reaction. A reaction peculiar to the individual.

Allergy. An altered reactivity. A reaction differing from the normal. An *allergen* is the substance which causes the abnormal reaction to occur. The term *antigen* implies a substance which stimulates the body to produce *antibodies.* It is a substance which is chemically different from the substances in our bodies and our bodies make chemical compounds which will unite with them. These compounds are so formed that they will unite only with the antigen which stimulated their production or one very similar to it. We say that the action of this substance is specific and call it an *antibody.*

An antigen which has a poisonous action is called a *toxin.* The antibody formed against it and which neutralizes it is called an *antitoxin.* Diphtheria antitoxin will neutralize diphtheria toxin but it will not have any effect on tetanus toxin. There are other antibodies which do not neutralize toxins but may cause bacteria to clump together, may cause precipitation of suspended substances or may cause dissolution of cells. These antibodies are also quite specific.

Reagin is the name applied to the antibody which is found in the blood and tissues of most allergic persons and is responsible for the reactions obtained to "skin tests." It is believed to be the antibody which causes the patient to be allergic and it reacts only with the substance, such as ragweed, feathers, or some foods, which causes its production.

Atopy (Greek, *atopia,* strangeness). A strange disease. Used interchangeably with allergy to describe certain forms of the disease as it affects human beings. An *atopen* is an allergen.

Sensitization. This, like antenna and clutch, is a borrowed word, adopted from photography. In the preparation of the photographic film, silver salts are treated with certain chemicals so that they become sensitive or sensitized to the action of sunlight. They then react differently on exposure to sunlight, as can be proved by the addition of more chemicals, in the process of photographic development. A *sensitized person* is one who will react differently, not necessarily to sunlight but to some special substance. The words sensitization and allergy are used interchangeably. A *sensitive person* is an allergic. A *sensitizer* is an allergen or antigen.

Anaphylaxis (Greek, *ana,* up, + *phylaxis,* protection). A lifting up of or taking away of protection. Removal of protection. The term is used to designate the changes occurring in animals who, artificially, have been made sensitive to some substance which previously was entirely innocuous. The term is used by some as interchangeable with allergy on the assumption that anaphylactic animals and allergic humans are suffering from the same condition. This is still a much argued question.

There is a group of terms frequently misused. To the patient, anything which is injected is either a serum or a vaccine. A *serum* is always derived from the blood of an animal and is given because it contains protective substances, antibodies, which have been manufactured by the living cells of the animal. Diphtheria antitoxin and tetanus antitoxin are examples. A *vaccine* is a suspension of the causative agent of the disease, such as a bacterium or a virus. Smallpox vaccine, typhoid vaccine, rabies vaccine are examples. An *extract* is a solution of certain parts of a plant or germ or other substance. Pollen extract or dust extract contains, in solution, the allergenic substance of pollen or dust.

Skin Tests. There are three methods commonly in use for doing these. One is a series of scratches which break the skin and, upon them, the application of a solution of an allergen. Or pin pricks may be made through a drop of extract, carrying a minute amount of the material into the skin. A much more sensitive method of testing is to inject into the skin a minute drop of the extract. This latter method is more sensitive than the others and may produce reactions which are missed by the other methods. However, this latter method may produce reactions of such intensity as to make the patient very ill, so it should not be used until the other methods have been tried first and found to give negative reactions. If a patient is sufficiently sensitive to give severe reaction on the injection testing, he will give a reaction to the scratch test, in which event he does not need the injection tests. If he shows no reaction to the scratch tests he will not show any dangerous reaction to the injection method.

Since the antibodies are supposed to be in the skin as well as in the blood, the purpose of the test is to get a minute amount of the allergen in contact with the antibodies. If a tiny amount of ragweed extract is placed in the skin of a patient sensitive to ragweed pollen, it should find the ragweed antibody there, and union of these two substances should produce a small, localized reaction characterized by swelling, redness, warmth, and usually itching. If the patient is sensitive only to ragweed then his skin should contain only antibodies for ragweed, and where other substances are introduced into the skin there is no antigen-antibody union and no reaction.

Unfortunately, in actual usage, the tests are not so perfect as the theory implies and have to be interpreted in the light of the patient's history.

Conjunctival Tests are done by placing a drop of an extract or the powdered material into the conjunctival sac. Changes consisting of redness, swelling, and weeping indicate a reaction.

A **Nasal Test** consists of the dropping, spraying, or inhaling of an extract or powder into the nose. A reaction consists of sneezing, a thin, watery nasal discharge and swelling of the nasal mucous membrane. These reactions have a limited usefulness but are sometimes more dependable than skin tests. All of these tests depend upon the presence of antibody in the tissues.

III

THE ALLERGIC CONSTITUTION

Allergy is not primarily an organic disease like tuberculosis, nephritis or Bright's disease, liver abscess or acute appendicitis, in which you can take out a certain organ and, examining it, find structural changes, with destruction of normal tissues due to the action of bacteria or other parasites or poisons. After an attack of hay fever, migraine or of urticaria has terminated, the tissues usually return completely to normal. Between attacks the victim is not conscious of any illness. The asthmatic may be quite normal during his intervals of freedom. It is only after the asthmatic paroxysms have lasted long or have been frequently repeated that secondary changes due to infection and other causes produce permanent damage. In this sense, allergy is not so much a disease as it is a temporary disturbance in the normal physiological mechanism, a reversible reaction which will return to normal when the cause has ceased to act.

The importance of controlling it before secondary changes have occurred is obvious.

Some persons are constituted differently from others. They respond to contact with environmental substances, whether these be foods eaten, pollen or dust inhaled, or things that come into contact with the skin, in a manner different from that of the majority of persons. They have "the allergic constitution." Doctors of the "idiosyncrasy" era called it the exudative diathesis, but "allergic constitution" is more up to date. The term implies, quite correctly, that the whole body participates in the reaction. This is true so far as we know, although only certain tissues react sufficiently to produce symptoms.

The Shock Tissues

The reactive regions are called shock tissues and involve especially the nose, the bronchi or air tubes in the lungs, the skin, and the stomach and intestines. Since the reacting tissue is primarily the blood vessel, then any tissue containing blood vessels can act as a shock tissue. And, while the tissues mentioned are the most frequent sites of reaction, we may see reactions anywhere in the body. There may be an involvement of the iris in the eye, in the internal ear, in the vessels in the meninges (the membranes surrounding the brain), or of the membranes lining the joints. Anyone who has spent years in the field of allergy has seen instances of these and many other involvements in areas which are usually not thought of as locations of allergic reactions.

It should be noted that these four shock tissues are situated at points where the body comes in contact with substances in the outside world. It is true even in the stomach and intestines. Food still present inside that long tube which extends downward from the mouth is not actually inside the body until after it has been digested and absorbed. Split a lead pencil lengthwise and remove the lead from the two little grooves running the length of the wood. Put the two sections of wood together and there is a long empty tube containing air. Although this tube of air is enveloped by the pencil it is not a part of the pencil. The pencil now has two sides, an outer side and an inner one, and the latter as well as the former is in contact with the outside world. Only if you were to bore a little hole in the wood, fill it with parts of the lead, and seal it over, would the lead be actually inside the pencil proper.

There are three things which you should remember, since they are important to an adequate understanding.

First, allergy is a general constitutional phenomenon which may involve almost any part of the body, espe-

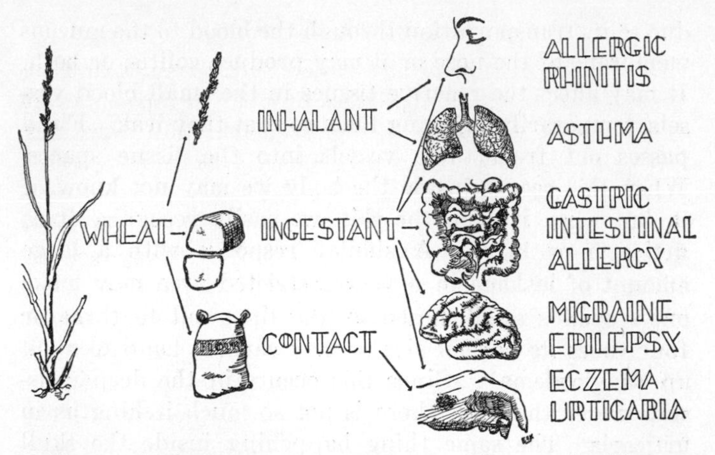

Different shock tissues may react even with a single allergen, depending in part on the mode of contact or exposure.

cially if enough of the allergen is absorbed into the blood to be transported wherever the blood goes.

Second, certain shock tissues are more likely to react than others. These are located at points of contact with the outer world and are therefore exposed to the allergen in much higher concentration than other tissues.

Third, these and other tissues are likely to react even though the contact may not be direct, provided enough of the allergenic excitant is carried to them through the blood. This is especially true in food allergy, since a local reaction in the stomach or intestines does not prevent continued absorption of the food.

Thus, one who inhales pollen develops hay fever or asthma. This is a matter of direct contact. One drinks milk and may or may not have indigestion, depending upon how reactive the shock tissue in the intestines happens to be, but may experience asthma from drinking milk, after this excitant has been absorbed into the blood and carried to the bronchi. An overdose of pollen extract given hypodermically may produce hay fever due to its transportation through the blood to the mucous membrane of the nose or it may produce colitis, or both. It may affect the reactive tissues in the small blood vessels, temporarily injuring them so that they leak. Fluid passes out from these vessels into the tissue spaces. When this occurs inside the body we may not know of it, but when it is in the skin we easily recognize it as urticaria or hives. A similar response with a large amount of leakage in a very restricted area may make one's eyelids swell closed or the lip swell to three or four times its normal size or may cause a hand to swell up (angioedema). Since this occurs in the deeper tissues under the skin, there is not so much itching as in urticaria. The same thing happening inside the skull may be responsible for migraine or sick headache. And now we come to a fourth point which should be remembered.

Fourth, not all shock tissues in a given person are necessarily reactive. One victim never has anything but asthma while another regularly manifests his allergy with attacks of colitis. Or one may have a reaction to one allergen in a certain tissue and to another allergen in a different tissue. Or one may have eczema as a child, lose it, and find it supplanted by asthma due to an entirely different allergen. And we have seen a patient with a summer dermatitis gradually lose it as hay fever, due to the same pollen, gradually replaced it.

There is some evidence that although allergy is a constitutional affair, sensitization to a given allergen may be localized in one shock tissue or another. Possibly it is just limited to this particular tissue or it may be that the reaction capacity is stronger here than in others. The only explanation we have for this phenomenon is that in the reacting tissues there is a high concentration of antibodies which unite with the allergen to produce the reaction. There are some antibodies elsewhere, as shown by the reaction in the skin test of a patient suffering from hay fever and whose symptoms are limited to the upper respiratory tract. Too, if a patient who has never shown any allergic manifestation except hay fever receives an overdose of the pollen, he not only has a severe attack of hay fever but may also develop asthma and hives and may be profoundly shocked. Whether this be true or not we may speak of specific sensitization in individual shock tissues. Thus, a woman always had migraine after eating celery. Celery caused no indigestion at all. But whenever she ate carrots she had attacks of colic, and no migraine at all.

Now, possibly, we are getting to where we can understand why different people react differently when sensitized to the same allergen or why a single person reacts variously with different allergens. It is a matter of these shock tissues. The tissue which bears the burden of the first and more concentrated contact with things from outside the body (extrinsic allergens) is more likely to react provided it has the reacting habit. If not, other shock tissues may react after absorption of the allergen and its transport to them through the blood. Here again it depends upon which ones have the trigger cocked—which are reactive—since it is not necessary that all shock tissues in a certain individual be in a reactive mood. Finally, and probably on account of local sensitization, one shock tissue may react to a given allergen while another reacts to others.

What Happens?

What actually happens when these shock tissues react? Allergists still argue among themselves about this. As we said earlier, many men think anaphylaxis in animals is the same thing as allergy in man. So they expect to find the same reactions in the human tissues in allergy as they find in animals with anaphylaxis. In animals the outstanding finding is the contraction of smooth or involuntary muscle. This does not refer to the voluntary muscle which we can move ourselves but to so-called involuntary or smooth muscle which is entirely free from the control of the will. It is the type of muscle that regulates the size of the pupils of the eyes and of the blood vessels, and which churns up food and forces it along the length of the intestinal tract. It is the chicken gizzard which we eat on Sunday and the intestinal muscle that goes into colicky cramps when we eat green apples.

There are similar circular bands of smooth muscle around the smaller bronchi—the air tubes deep down in the lungs—which regulate the amount of air entering the lungs themselves. At autopsies which had been done on people who had chronic asthma, a definite thickening of the bronchial muscle has been found which has been interpreted to mean that the greater amount of muscle has resulted from the frequent contractions, and the increased thickening decreases the size of the tube and so causes the difficult breathing to become continuous. There is no question as to the finding of increased amount of bronchial musculature in these cases; there is considerable argument as to whether this is the cause of the dyspnea or the result of it.

There is general agreement as to the importance of increased capillary permeability. This means that the cells lining the smallest blood vessels, the capillaries which connect the ends of the arteries with the beginnings of the veins, are damaged so that they cannot keep fluid, as they should, from pouring out into the tissues. They become more sieve-like and the blood pressure forces fluid to leak out. This explains hives, angioneurotic edema (the larger localized swellings previously mentioned), and weeping eczema. It explains the swelling and obstruction in the little

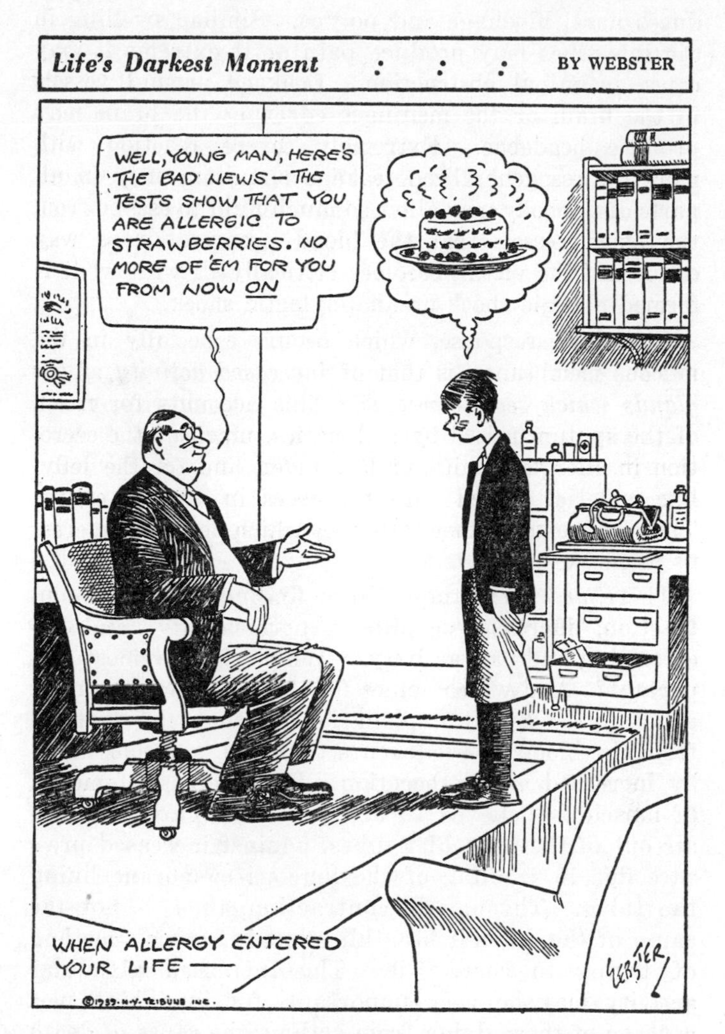

(Published by permission of *New York Herald Tribune.*)

bronchi or bronchioles. Swelling of the mucous membranes in the nose due to fluid transudation produces nasal blockage and polyps. Similar swelling in the intestines may produce pain or if extreme it may cause intestinal obstruction. Leakage around vessels in the brain or the meninges covering the brain may produce headache. Extremely severe reaction with more or less generalized leakage simultaneously in all parts of the body may allow so much fluid to escape from the blood vessels that the blood pressure drops way down and the victim becomes critically ill with what is termed allergic shock or anaphylactic shock.

The third response, which occurs especially in the mucous membranes, is that of *increased activity of the glands which secrete mucus.* This accounts for much of the sputum raised by asthmatics, much of the secretion in allergic rhinitis or hay fever, and for the jelly-like material passed with the feces in mucous colitis. There are certain other responses which need not interest us just now.

There are then, these three findings: muscle contraction, increased capillary permeability, and increased glandular activity. Which is the most important? And which comes first? In asthma the most generally accepted explanation is that the leakage from the blood vessels occurs first and is accompanied by increased gland secretion. The increased amount of muscle is believed to be due to the effort to push air out of the bronchial tubes, against increased pressure due to swelling of the mucous membrane lining the tubes. The muscle contraction, then, is not the cause of the difficult breathing but is nature's method of trying to correct it. The increased glandular activity may be very important, for in a high percentage of those dying from asthma the cause of death seems to be the blocking of the tubes by the tough, tenacious secretion.

Although allergic reactions may occur in different parts of the body, they are fundamentally the same. The difference in symptoms is due to the location and the kind of tissue involved. There is no fundamental difference between hay fever and asthma; the difference in symptoms is due entirely to the fact that in the one instance the reaction is in the nose while in the other it is in the bronchial tubes.

Theories to Explain Allergy

Now we know why allergics react differently even among themselves and can explain why the symptoms are such as they are. But we don't yet know what chemical or other sort of changes occur in the body during the process of becoming allergic to a given substance. What has happened that makes this person respond in an altered manner? There is an answer, in fact there have been many answers suggested, no two of which agree altogether and none of which explain the situation to complete satisfaction. Some of them are very complicated. Certainly none of them is simple. For the present discussion a simple explanation is most desirable. So, I shall have to leave out a lot of *ifs* and *buts* and *howevers,* and warn the reader that the explanation given is merely to facilitate an understanding of what *might* be happening. To make it more comprehensible, although less accurate, I shall explain what might be taking place, by means of a simile, comparing the human body, with its myriad of living cells, to a great city or state, in which each person corresponds to a cell in the body. Let us, for fun, call this democracy the *State of Allergy.*

The unit of life in the living body is the cell. The body was started from the union of two cells, no more. These reproduced and continued to reproduce until there were billions of them all pretty well attached to each other. The tremendous number of cells in the human body may be conceived when we realize that a drop of blood no larger than an ordinary pinhead contains about five million red blood cells. The body is made up almost entirely of living, working cells, and structures that they have built for self-protection, such as bone and cartilage or gristle, tendons, skin, hair, etc. Water and minerals help keep these structures in continuity.

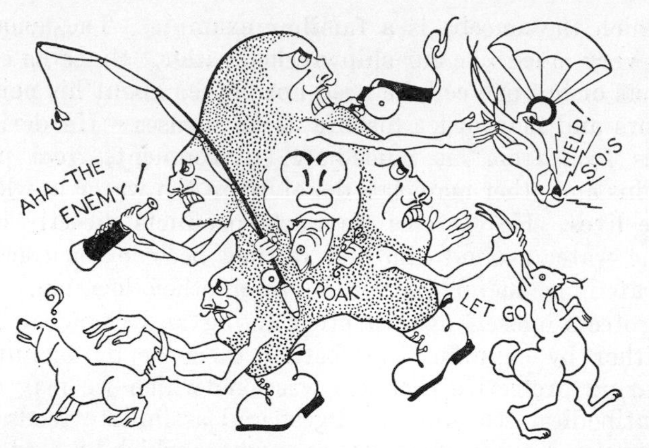

An Amoeba, in Search of Food and Armed Against Enemies

IV

THE STATE OF ALLERGY

A shipwrecked sailor on a deserted island would find that he must procure and prepare his own food, build his own shelter, arrange effective protection against possible wild beasts or poisonous reptiles or insects, and make some sort of substitute for clothing. The absence of sanitary facilities would not upset him greatly since there is no one near, to be offended. If his carelessness eventually offends himself, he may move to another locality.

If he finds living sources of danger in his environment, he will make implements with which to protect himself. These weapons will be different, depending upon the nature of the enemy, whether it be mosquito, hornet, snake, tiger or vultures. If we were to visit our castaway's island, we should be able to determine the nature of the enemy merely by examining the defensive weapons.

The lowest form of animal life which we can observe through an ordinary microscope is the protozoan, of which the amoeba is a familiar example. The amoeba is very much like our shipwrecked sailor. Since he consists of but one cell, he need not bother about his neighbors and may order his life as he pleases. He derives his food from his immediate environment, from proteins and other materials dissolved in the water in which he lives. He excretes his waste products directly into the water around him and if they become too concentrated, he merely moves on to another location. He protects himself against other living and chemical foes either by engulfing and eating them or by manufacturing protective chemical weapons which we may call antibodies. In order to digest and assimilate foods, he secretes digestive ferments or enzymes which break down the more complex food proteins, fats and carbohydrates into simpler compounds which may be absorbed, just as the human being does in the alimentary canal.

This single cell can move, breathe, eat, excrete, and fight.

In the course of evolution, the earliest amoebae and other protozoa discovered advantages in a community existence, with a larger number of cells attached to each other. As various species have developed the number remaining attached increased until, in man, it is enormous.

Just as the shipwrecked sailor would have to modify his mode of living if he found himself in a civilized community, the cells must adjust themselves to new environmental conditions. The sailor need no longer bother about provisions, since there are groups of persons whose business it is to import food products, making them available for the community. He need not protect himself against recognized enemies since there are especially equipped soldiers and policemen whose duty it is to attend to this function. He may now no longer deposit his waste in the streets. It is safely removed from the community in conduits built especially for this purpose.

Let us study this community of human cells which we have termed the State of Allergy. We find that the sailor's deserted island has now developed into a large industrial country, long and narrow, through the length of which runs a tremendous canal, down which barges are floating, bringing food supplies right in to the center of the country. Here they tie up at docks and unload their supplies, which are stored in storehouses, to be used as needed.

The country has a seashore frontier, called Skin. Throughout this outer boundary, there is a layer of specialized cells whose duty it is to prevent invasion from without. Figuratively they constitute a protective wall somewhat akin to the Great Wall of China. Behind the wall are soldiers, the mobile leukocytes or white blood cells which move freely, just like amoebae do, and one of whose functions is to engulf and destroy any bacteria, enemies invading the country from without.

Wireless communication with foreign States is maintained through two great sets of receiving stations named Eyes and Ears. The latter are remotely located, deep-set in the mountain fastness, almost completely protected from invasion. The eye receiving stations are right on the beach, badly exposed, but they have a protective camouflage which may be thrown over them. It looks just like the great wall.

The broadcasting station is located at the entrance to the canal. Here also one finds a double system of locks or protective gates. On each side of the grand canal there are forts, filled with the little soldiers, and named Tonsils. Air is brought into the community through a series of ducts, somewhat like those built into the walls of modern air-conditioned buildings. There are protective barricades in these ducts. The ciliated epithelium of the nose actually has little fine microscopic brushes which sweep foreign matter out toward the entrance. Similar sweepers are found in the lower ducts. If irritating material enters these air passages, there is a protective mechanism that works somewhat like an exhaust explosion. It is called a Sneeze. The entrance to the inner series of ducts is protected by a trap door, the Epiglottis, and a pair of curtains which may be drawn tightly together. These are called Vocal Cords. If irritating substances manage to pass these protections, little muscles in the smallest ducts contract down, to protect further against foreign invasion. Parcels of oxygen delivered into the warehouse of the lungs are carried through the streets and highways of the community, the blood vessels, by little delivery boys, the red blood cells, to those cells needing this commodity.

Now let us follow one of the barges as it passes along the grand canal, and observe what happens to the supplies being brought into the country. Soon the channel broadens out into a large lagoon named Stomach and here the barge is boarded by customs inspectors. They commence sorting the material being imported, an important piece of work which will be continued by others farther along the canal. If they find harmful materials or dangerous enemies on the barge, they are likely to send them back, throwing them out of the State. Sometimes, however, the inspectors fail to recognize harmful materials or living enemies.

The barge passes out of the lagoon. Farther on, it is tied up alongside a pier where its contents are unloaded. In the warehouses the large cases are undone, their contents are sorted and sent on their way, each to its proper destination, being carried chiefly along the highways mentioned above.

As we pass out of the distributing centers, the warehouses, into the highways we find a very busy little nation indeed. The little red messenger boys must carry their parcels to every living member of the community and they are tumbling over each other in their haste to make delivery and to carry back some of the parcels of carbon dioxide, no longer needed and destined for export. We run into the little white policemen here and there, everywhere. They patrol highways and are ready at a signal to squeeze out of the blood vessels, between the working cells, to arrest any foreign prowler.

In this nation every individual works. You never saw such a busy community. As we go along the highway we reach great factory buildings, each making some special type of material to be used by others in the community. For this purpose they utilize the raw materials brought in on the barges or through the air ducts, which are delivered to the proper factories on the endless conveyor-belt system of the blood stream. One of these factories is called Liver, another Pancreas, another the Thyroid. There are others. Waste materials are delivered onto the conveyor system, sent to special plants whose function it is to remove them from the conveyor, transferring them to the sewage system for ultimate disposal.

The communication system is remarkably efficient. There is a telephone system of Nerves which constantly conveys messages to the headquarters of the governing body, the Brain, reporting the state of the nation. The Nerves carry, in return, general orders and special orders governing activities to be carried out even in remotest parts of the nation. Then there are messengers running up and down the streets, Hormones, carrying communications from certain factories to others, telling them when to speed up work or to shut down.

Home Defense

We find a very interesting arrangement for protection of the community against enemies. The shipwrecked sailor, like the amoeba, had to provide his own protection. But when the population became metropolitan, certain workers were assigned this function. While, as we have seen, policemen are here and there in the streets and in the factory buildings, preventing internal disorder, there are others, soldiers, not necessarily the little leukocytic policemen but other types of cells, stationed at strategic places on the frontiers, whose duty it is to resist invasion. They appear to be especially active in those localities that we have spoken of as the allergic shock tissues, the nose, bronchi, skin and gastro-intestinal mucous membrane. The primary function of these tissues is that of protection. When working normally they do this. A foreign body such as dust in the nose causes sneezing and watery secretion, designed to wash it away. Irritating material inhaled into the bronchi causes cough, an increased secretion of mucus, and if these reactions are very pronounced, as in heavy smokers, one may even detect actual asthmatic wheezing. Harmful substances entering the alimentary canal are likely to be vomited or removed later with the ensuing diarrhea. Irritants applied to the skin produce a protective reaction in which serum leaks out of the blood vessels and surrounds the living cells, presumably to protect them. If the irritation is low-grade but long-continued, this develops into weeping eczema. If more severe and more acute, as in a burn, fluid accumulates to such a degree as to produce a blister. Fundamentally these are protective reactions.

Since there are certain groups of cells stationed more or less as sentries, other cells within the body need not bother about protection. As with humans, they lose much of their ability to protect themselves. Harmful foreign substances are kept out of the body in so far as possible, but when they do enter, they find cells which they can injure much more easily than the more primitive cells. In the same manner these cells have lost much of their ability to digest food which might be available in their environment. The chief characteristic of the community of cells is that of specialization. Certain groups of the workers have the function of contracting. These are the Muscle cells. Others manufacture and secrete substances into the blood. Still others, the Nerves, conduct nervous impulses. Workers along the banks of the grand canal are trained to digest and they do this for the entire community.

Application to Allergy

We are now in a position to discuss in terms of our allegory what *might* be happening when a person becomes sensitized. Citizens of the State of Allergy are living in what to them is a very pleasant environment, with a nearly constant temperature and climate. The workers carry on their duties, bathed in a fluid which is remarkably constant and nonirritating in character. The cells on the frontiers see to it that under normal conditions harmful or irritating substances are excluded from the community.

But occasionally such substances slip unnoticed past the border patrols. Whether this material which enters the highways and byways of the principality be some unaccustomed drug or a living germ or dead vaccine, horse serum or a food protein which should normally have been at least partially digested before admittance, these are new and strange substances which should not be allowed in the immediate environment of the workers. Being strangers they are enemies. In fact, being chemicals they tend to attach themselves to the workers, actually injuring the latter. Under such circumstances what will the workers do to protect themselves? They will manufacture some sort of rudimentary weapons with which they may combat the invading enemy. By means of laboratory tests we can demonstrate that such substances actually appear in the blood after such an invasion. We call them antibodies or reagins (see definitions, Chapter II). It takes the workers some time to make their weapons. Research has shown that at least ten days are required.

As with the shipwrecked sailor and the amoeba, different types of weapons are made for different types of enemies.

If after the ten-day interval the enemy again invades, quite a fight ensues. One of the by-products of the battle, probably emanating from wounded worker cells, is a chemical substance known as histamine. This is found to be especially abundant near the site of a reaction, probably is the cause of the dilation of the blood vessels and their subsequent leaking, and may be carried through the blood to remote parts. We might look upon histamine, as it is being carried through the blood, as a series of messages reporting that all is not well. These messages reach the frontier outposts, the shock tissues, which promptly go into action, using their antibodies with the purpose of preventing any more of the enemy (antigen, allergen) from entering the country. The trouble is that everyone is excited. As a consequence the frontier forces become too active, almost we might say going into spasms to prevent further invasion. This overactivity results in the common allergic symptoms previously described.

In this instance, the enemy is already within the country and there may be no additional forces trying to effect entry through the skin, lungs or intestinal tract. The protective shock tissues in these three localities may go into action just as violently as though there were, on the assumption that since the enemy is already within the boundaries, more might try to enter.

Depending upon the nature of the allergen and the amount of antibody weapons available in the different shock tissues, symptoms will appear in one or another of these localities. In general they are more likely to occur at the point of entrance of the allergen. Thus one who is allergic to house dust, and inhales house dust, is more likely to have asthma than colitis, although the reverse may occur. Foods are more likely than other allergens to cause symptoms in shock tissues remote from the point of entrance, probably because it has been shown that, normally, food is not always completely digested before absorption into the blood. When the allergen is introduced through the skin as with a hypodermic needle, any or all of the shock tissues may become involved. In any case, however, the protective reaction is out of proportion to the amount of local excitation. The reaction is a purposeful one, but since it is very much overdone, even to the point of causing discomfort, we may speak of it as purposelessly executed.

We may think of epinephrine (Adrenalin), ephedrine, and certain other drugs as relieving the symptoms by virtue of bringing about a constriction of the blood vessels and preventing further leakage. The fluid which has already leaked from the vessels is absorbed and the tissue reverts to its normal state. The antihistaminic drugs are believed to act by preventing the action of histamine which was the cause of the capillary leakage. They supply the governing balance which prevents the shock tissues from overreacting. Epinephrine is normally present in the body and is one of the hormones or messengers that are carried to different tissues to direct them as to how to carry on their work.

Back to Earth

This explanation of the State of Allergy is certainly not what one would term scientific, but since none of the scientific explanations has been universally accepted and since our allegory is actually based upon the known facts and upon the two most generally accepted theories, and since it involves no highly technical terminology, the writer presents it in the hope that it will enable the reader to derive a general idea of what might be happening in the allergic person.

Certain fundamental facts of allergy become apparent. In the development of an allergic state, the person originally is not sensitized. He will not become sensitized to a given allergen until after that allergen has entered the tissues of the body, theoretically causing damage. Thereafter the tissues gradually become sensitized. This process requires at least ten days. At times it is much longer. After sensitization has occurred, reagins may be shown to be present in the blood. Thereafter, if the antigen again enters the tissues, the reaction is prompt, sometimes almost explosive, producing the symptoms of allergic disease. During the reaction histamine accumulates in the blood and tissues, more abundantly in shock tissues than elsewhere.

The antibodies or defensive weapons are specific, that is, they are different for each different type of invader. They may be identified by blood tests or skin tests. This is what is done in the familiar procedure of "skin testing.''

Questions and Answers

Q. You have given us an explanation of what happens when one becomes sensitized. But you haven't told us why some persons become allergic while others do not.

A. We really don't know precisely why some become sensitized to substances in their immediate environment while others do not. This will be touched on in a measure in the next chapter. There is, however, one clearly recognized factor which appears to predetermine one's susceptibility to sensitization. This is heredity. *Allergy is an hereditary disease,* being transmitted apparently by male and female alike. What one inherits is not a specific sensitization to some particular allergen such as ragweed pollen or wheat, nor a specific type of response such as asthma or migraine. Instead one inherits the *tendency to become sensitized* to substances. What those substances are to be and how one will react to them, what shock tissue will be involved, depend more upon the manner and nature of allergenic exposures after birth. There is an old tradition that ''asthma tends to run in families'' and a similar one regarding migraine. However, other allergic symptoms are probably as common, taking the family group as a whole.

Q. I am allergic and so far as I know there is no history of allergy in my family. How then can it be hereditary?

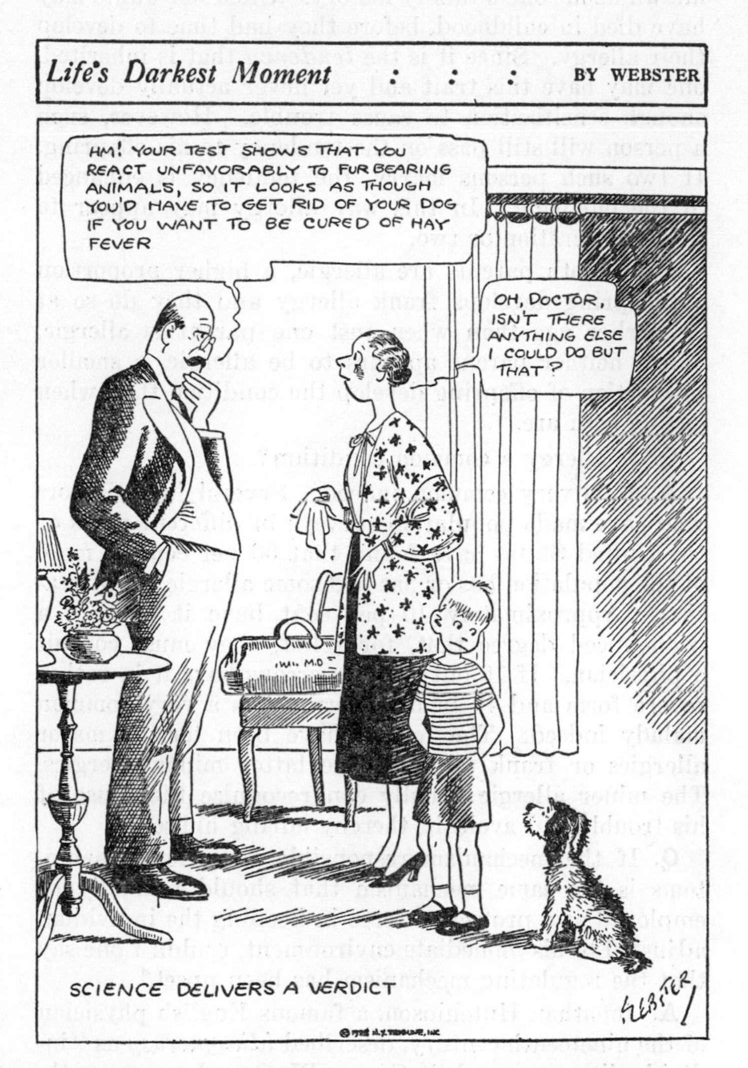

(Published by permission of *New York Herald Tribune.*)

A. Sometimes one doesn't know all that there is to be known about one's family history. Uncles or aunts may have died in childhood, before they had time to develop their allergy. Since it is the *tendency* that is inherited, one may have this trait and yet never actually develop enough sensitization to cause trouble. However, such a person will still pass on the tendency to his offspring. If two such persons marry, the tendency is enhanced in the offspring. In this way allergy may appear to skip a generation or two.

When both parents are allergic, a higher proportion of offspring develops frank allergy and they do so at an earlier age than when just one parent is allergic. When neither parent appears to be allergic, a smaller proportion of offspring develop the condition than when one or both are.

Q. Is allergy a common condition?

A. It is very common indeed. Several investigators who have made population surveys in different parts of the United States have found that 50 per cent or more of the population has or has had some allergic manifestation. Approximately 10 per cent have it to such a pronounced degree that, for relief, they must consult a physician. If 10 out of 100 persons have it in rather severe form and 40 in mild form, it is a very common malady indeed. The former have been termed major allergics or frank allergics, the latter minor allergics. The minor allergic usually can recognize the cause of his trouble and avoid it, thereby curing himself.

Q. If the mechanism responsible for allergic symptoms is the same mechanism that should normally be employed as a protective force in keeping the individual adjusted to his immediate environment, couldn't one say that the regulating mechanism has been upset?

A. Jonathan Hutchinson, a famous English physician of the nineteenth century, described *idiosyncrasy* as "individuality gone mad." George W. Gray has very aptly described allergy as "protection gone wild."

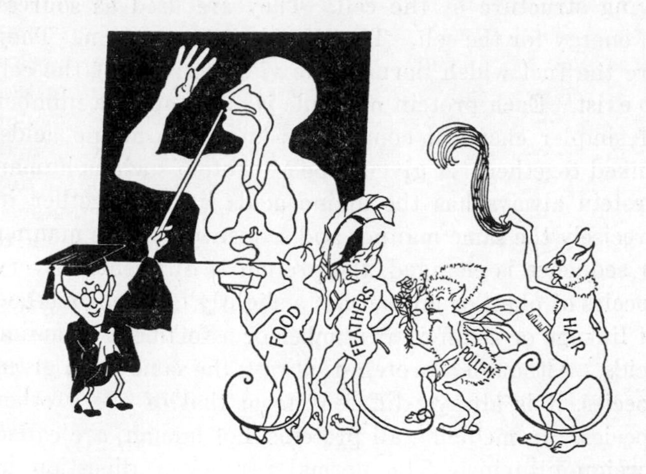

Allergens, Preparing to Invade the State of Allergy

V

THE ENEMY—ALLERGENS

We have rather given the impression in the last chapter that almost any type of foreign substance entering the body may produce allergic sensitization. This appears to be almost true, although there are certain kinds which are more likely to do so than others.

Protein

Chief among these is foreign protein. The basic structure of every living cell is protein. The living part of every plant and animal is protein. When we eat meat or egg white the chief substance ingested is protein. There is some protein in nearly all natural foods. There are also carbohydrates, starches, and fats but these three groups of materials are not, like protein, built into the living structure of the cell. They are used as sources of energy for the cell. They enable it to carry on. They are the fuel which permits the vital activity of the cell to exist. Each protein molecule is made up of a number of simpler chemical compounds known as amino acids, linked together. A given type of protein such as human protein always has the amino acids linked together in precisely the same manner and sequence. If the manner or sequence is changed, the protein is different. Every species of plant or animal has a slightly different method of linkage or a different number or assortment of amino acids. Although a protein is always the same for a given species, it is always different from that of every other species. In medicine all proteins, not human, are called foreign proteins. The normal process of digestion in the alimentary canal breaks the foreign proteins into their constituent amino acids and the latter are absorbed, to be used by the living cells of the body for the purpose of building more of their own protein. According to the prevailing theories of digestion, foreign protein as such seldom enters the tissues and the blood stream. If it does, it damages the body cells chemically, as a result of which the latter become sensitized to it. If at some later time the foreign protein again enters the body, allergic symptoms ensue.

This has been seen occasionally, for example, after the injection of immune sera, usually from horses. The first injection produces no symptoms, but if a second injection is given a few months later, one may react with hives, asthma, allergic shock or other anaphylactic symptoms. One may even have hives after the first injection. This is known as serum sickness. It occurs about ten days after the serum injection and is due to the fact that some horse serum is still present in the blood, not yet excreted or destroyed, at the time when sensitization has taken place. The cells, having perfected their weapons of defense, attack the small amount of serum still present. This form of serum sickness is very troublesome but never serious.

Human plasma given in the treatment of disease, as in transfusion, will not cause allergy because the protein is identical to that already present. Some allergic reactions have followed transfusions of human blood, due usually to the fact that the donor had recently eaten some food to which the recipient was already allergic or to the fact that the donor was allergic to something which the recipient had just eaten.

Other Allergens

Early investigators in anaphylaxis believed that only proteins could produce sensitization. This included not only foods and inhaled substances such as house dust, feather dust, pollens, and horse dander but also bacteria. In the course of time it developed that drugs such as quinine, aspirin, arsphenamine and iodine could sensitize. Since all of the theories were based upon the premise of protein sensitization, the suggestion was made that these chemicals combined with the human protein in the circulating blood, to form a new and different protein which acts as a foreign protein. Much experimental work appears to have confirmed this belief.

Next it developed that substances in contact with the skin, apparently not entering the body at all, may produce local sensitization with resulting dermatitis or eczema. Very diverse things were found to do this. Soap, lipstick, shoe polish, mascara, formaldehyde, clothing, furs, medicines, ointments, different kinds of sawdust, paint, synthetic chemicals, plants (including not only poison ivy but such harmless leaves as maple and elm), and even simple chemical elements such as nickel were found capable of producing allergic dermatitis in susceptible individuals.

We can still postulate a combination of these substances with body protein, the protein of the cells in the skin itself. This has not yet been proved.

Finally a new group of allergic excitants was recognized in what has come to be termed physical allergy, allergic reaction to the effect of heat, cold, sunlight, and physical effort. Since one can scarcely hypothesize a combination of heat or cold with human protein to make a new protein, we are forced to believe that, in these people, the temperature changes either change the body protein so that it becomes, in effect, a foreign protein, or that there may be antibodies in the patient which are active only when there is some change in the body temperature, or that there may be histamine liberated without an antigen-antibody reaction.

It was stated above that some substances are more likely to produce sensitization than others, that they are more highly allergenic. What factors determine this allergenic capacity?

There are two basic factors, first the nature of the allergen and, second, the degree of the inherited tendency in the individual.

Nature of the Allergen

Foreign protein leads the list of substances likely to produce sensitization. Since it is present in all living things, the list may be very long indeed. Fortunately, however, the body is normally well protected against the admittance of undigested protein into the system. Foreign protein is in its most highly allergenic state when it enters the system without any previous digestion or treatment, as after hypodermic or intravenous injection. Fortunately, with the exception of therapeutic sera, this rarely becomes necessary. Even among proteins there is a difference in allergenic capacity, some having more than others. We do not know precisely why, but there is evidence suggesting that the more foreign it is, the more likely it will be to sensitize. Thus it is easier to sensitize a person to guinea pig serum than to beef serum. In view of the fact that most of us eat beef nearly every day, we have adjusted or have acclimatized ourselves to it. It is not as foreign as guinea pig protein, to which we are rarely exposed.

In dealing with pollens we often state that some are more toxic than others. This is not a proper use of the word "toxic" which means poisonous, for if a pollen were truly toxic it should affect everyone which, of course, it does not do. There are some pollens which are more difficult to use in treatment because they so often cause reactions even with small increments of dosage. Marsh elder pollen, for example, has to be handled with great caution while ragweed pollen does not require nearly so much care. But neither of these is truly toxic. We can say that one is a better sensitizer than the other but why or how, we do not know.

This is a vaguely understood factor, in the allergen itself. Pine pollen is very abundant in appropriate sections but rarely causes sensitization. If a major allergic were exposed to the same quantity of pine and ragweed pollen for the same length of time, he would be much more likely to become sensitized to ragweed.

Susceptibility of the Host

The preceding statements apply more especially to the minor allergic, the person who has only occasional symptoms, the cause of which he can usually recognize. He is relatively insusceptible and consequently becomes sensitized only to the more highly foreign substances, if we may use this term, to substances with which he establishes only occasional contact. Among the foods, for example, he will become allergic to those which he eats only on occasion, such as watermelon, onion, oyster, clam, lobster, strawberries, cabbage, pork.

The major allergics, those comprising the 10 per cent of the population previously mentioned, those possessing heavy allergic inheritance, not only become sensitized to occasional substances but also to substances in their daily or regular environment, such as wheat, egg, milk, beef, coffee, house dust, feathers and the like. One might say that they are so highly allergic that they cannot acclimatize themselves to their normal environment. Since they are exposed daily or at frequent intervals to the allergens responsible for symptoms, they are unable to recognize them as offending substances and must therefore be tested with extracts of them in order to determine the offenders.

This concept of major and minor allergies does not, however, explain why one person becomes sensitive to wheat which he eats daily and another becomes sensitive to ragweed pollen to which he is exposed for about six weeks each year.

Intensity of Exposure

The greater the quantity of the substance to which one is exposed or the longer the duration of the expôsure, the more is there likelihood of consequent sensitization. This is true for both minor and major allergics. Only 10 per cent of persons receiving approximately 10 c.c. of horse serum become sensitized thereto, while 90 per cent of those receiving 100 c.c. or more do so. A minor allergic is more likely to become sensitized to chocolate if at some time he eats too much chocolate candy. Chocolate in moderation might never have produced trouble. The grass pollen season is longer than the ragweed season but, in ragweed sections, there is much more ragweed pollen in the air than grass pollen during their respective seasons. There is consequently much more sensitization to ragweed than to the grasses.

This has an important bearing on food allergies. Wheat, milk, and egg are usually used more frequently and in larger amounts than other foods, and they cause more allergic reactions than all other foods combined. It can be said, as a generalization, that people become sensitive to the foods which they use the most. Since people usually eat the most of things they like the best, allergists often state that, "We spend our days taking the joy out of people's lives." A person who has frequent, outspoken manifestations of allergy is seldom relieved by taking from his diet foods which he cares little for and seldom eats.

Other Factors

There are undoubtedly many other factors which play a part in determining to what one will become sensitized. If three persons eat wheat, egg, and milk every day, why does one become sensitized to wheat, another to egg, and the third to milk? The answer is not forthcoming. There is evidence that a "stomach upset" may predispose to the absorption of incompletely digested protein. Theoretically this should increase the tendency to sensitization to some food being eaten at the time of the upset. Other factors such as constipation, fatigue, intercurrent infection, etc., may play a part in determining sensitization. I have said that we do not inherit sensitization to some particular substance. However, an infant may be born sensitized to chocolate, egg or milk, something which he has never eaten. The circulation of the blood of the unborn child is fairly closely connected with that of the mother, and experimental study has shown that a child may be exposed through this mechanism to allergens which have entered the mother's circulation. There is some evidence that pregnant mothers who develop abnormal cravings for certain foods, eating them to excess, may sensitize their infants thereto.

If a person is to become sensitive to a certain food or pollen, what determines when this will occur? No one knows. Some allergists think sensitization will occur early if there is an inherited tendency and possibly much later if there is no evidence of heredity. But why should a farmer who breathes ragweed pollen every fall develop hay fever for the first time when he is 74 years old? Or why should one become asthmatic at the age of sixty from milk which he had drunk all his life? This does not depend on inheritance, or to change in the amount or character of the allergen to which the patient is exposed. Evidently some change in the patient's body takes place at this time but why or how we do not know.

Summary

Summarizing, we may say that, given sufficiently intensive exposure, a predisposed person may become allergic to almost any environmental substances; some of these are more highly allergenic than others; the more unfamiliar or the more foreign the substance, the greater the probability of high antigenicity; and a person with a heavy inherited predisposition may become sensitized even to substances which might be considered as a part of his natural or normal daily environment.

Questions and Answers

Q. Does a person usually become sensitized to only one allergen?

A. Single sensitizations do occur, especially among the minor allergics, but multiple sensitizations are the rule even with them. Not only may one be allergic to several foods but also to foods or ingestant allergens, to inhalant and contact or skin allergens.

Q. What is the largest number of substances to which a single person may be allergic?

A. It is theoretically possible to become sensitive to every food. As a matter of fact, we seldom see persons who are actually clinically sensitive to more than a few things, as may be shown by the relief obtained by the removal of these few foods from the diet. Sometimes long lists may be made of those foods which are thought to cause positive skin reaction, but actual use of the foods will show that few are the cause of symptoms.

Most food allergics are sensitized to more than one food, but not to so many that the necessary dietary restrictions will prevent them from obtaining ample nourishment, including sufficient vitamins, in the restricted diet. Sometimes this requires the addition of new foods not customarily eaten by the individual (see Chapter XI).

Q. Are skin tests reliable for determining the causative allergens?

A. When doing a skin test we are actually reproducing the allergic reaction in miniature form. With a scalpel or needle we penetrate the protective barrier of the skin and insert a very minute quantity of the suspected allergen directly in the tissues. The miniature local positive reaction (a single hive) is a localized replica of what happens in the illness. A positive reaction indicates an allergic response. It does not however necessarily indicate that the particular test substance is responsible for the present trouble. The remark has been made that the positive skin reaction is an historical landmark, indicating either past trouble, present trouble or potential future trouble. In short, one does not necessarily have trouble from everything that gives a positive reaction.

Not all positive reactions are true positives. We may encounter false positive reactions, usually the result of some irritating substance in the test material. Some allergists designate all positive reactions which cannot be shown to be responsible for symptoms at the time of study as false positives. Furthermore, there may be false negative reactions. A substance known to cause trouble may react negatively by skin test. This may be due to the fact that the test material is too weak or otherwise defective or it may be due to a lack of antibodies in the skin. It is assumed, though not proved, that one may have asthma from the presence of large amounts of antibodies in the bronchial mucous membrane but there may be no skin reaction because there are too few antibodies there. One hesitates to accept this explanation in the face of the fact that skin tests are notoriously fallible in urticaria which is an allergic reaction in the skin. Other theories could be presented but they would only add to the confusion.

In some allergic conditions, notably urticaria and eczema, we may frequently get negative reactions to foods which we may definitely show to be the cause of the condition. Why this should occur and why it should occur more frequently in these than in other conditions we do not know. This may add a great deal to the difficulty of the diagnosis.

In spite of the fact that skin tests are not 100 per cent reliable, the procedure is the best available objective or laboratory method for diagnosis. The physician realizes the possibility or indeed probability in each case of a certain proportion of false negative and false positive reactions and, as we shall see, he takes the necessary steps toward their ultimate recognition.

Q. Is there any danger of producing new sensitizations by performing skin tests? Will this artificial introduction of foreign substances cause sensitization to them?

A. Theoretically, the answer should be yes. As a matter of practical experience we may definitely say no. Doctors have intentionally produced sensitization to guinea pig serum by skin testing human beings several times in succession at weekly intervals. A certain proportion of persons immunized against diphtheria by injections of toxin-antitoxin become sensitized to horse serum. This sensitization, however, seems to be limited to the skin and does not mean that symptoms will develop after use of the method. As is probably true with all sensitizations, this is not permanent but gradually disappears. It should be noted that this has been done only with extremely foreign substances such as guinea pig and horse sera. A series of tests at weekly intervals was required even with them. Similar attempts to sensitize the common allergens such as house dust, orris root, and pollens have failed.

If a person were skin tested once a week for a period of several months, always with the same allergen or series of allergens, it might be possible to produce sensitization. Occasional testing as is done in routine allergic therapy does not sensitize. The amount of material used is too small and the reaction is too localized. Treatment with extracts of pollen or dust has been carried on over months or even years without any evidence of sensitizing the patient.

Q. Isn't it possible for a person to react to cooking odors?

A. The odor of frying food often causes asthma in susceptible individuals. Certain perfumes may do likewise. In other words we might say that persons can be allergic to smells.

This is not as far fetched as it might at first glance appear. French investigators have shown that odors, such as those from perfumes and other scents, are actually due to the presence of minute particles of matter, carried through the air to their destinations. In this case the destination is the mucous membrane of the nose or bronchi.

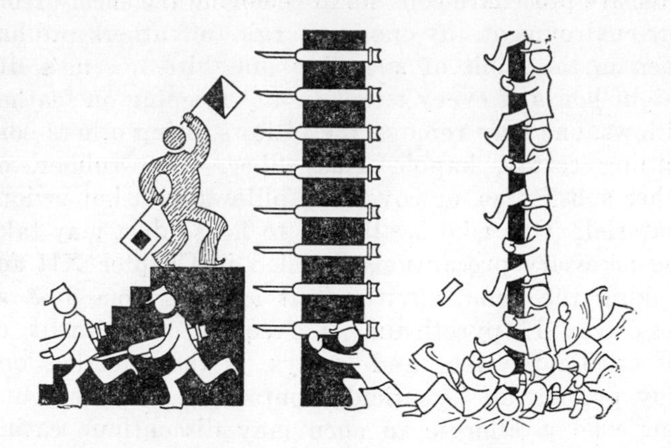

Excitement at the Firehouse; Antibodies Arming for Combat

VI

DEFENSE OF THE REALM—METHODS OF COMBATING SENSITIZATION

Up to the present the discussion of our problem may well appear rather gloomy. If a sensitized person must, thereafter, avoid the offending allergen; if sensitization is multiple and as time goes on he is likely to become sensitized to an increasing number of substances; and if some of these are substances which cannot be avoided, the outlook would appear to be that, as time goes on, the situation will become increasingly difficult and symptoms more persistent. In many instances this is true if no treatment is given. Fortunately, however, allergic treatment provides a method for breaking this vicious circle.

Offensive

The enemy having been identified, what may we do about it? Our attack may be offensive or defensive. The offensive procedure consists in removing the enemy from our environment. If one is allergic to feathers and has been in the habit of spending one-third of one's life (eight hours of every twenty-four) sleeping on feather pillows, one may remove the pillows, using others containing cotton, kapok, glass fiber, foam rubber, or other substitutes, or cover the pillows with impervious material. One who is allergic to house dust may take the necessary precautions detailed in Chapter XII for making the home environment as free from dust as possible. If pyrethrum, a frequent constituent of insecticide powders and sprays, is the offender, one may procure an insecticide containing no pyrethrum. One who is allergic to corn may discontinue eating corn and corn products. The victim of pollen allergy may live in an air-conditioned room equipped with a pollen filter. He who is allergic to dog hair may give away his dog.

Defensive

The defensive measures overlap the offensive ones just mentioned. They are of two general types. The first is the removal of ourselves from the environment in which the enemy exists. This may consist of moving to a part of the country in which a certain plant does not grow, or changing occupation or even just moving from the country to the city. One may go to the seashore during a pollen season or give up dairy farming. Or move to a large city where the amount of pollen in the air is low. These methods constitute a "strategic retreat." The second procedure is that of desensitization, a process which might be described as somewhat akin to that of acclimatization or adjustment of the tissues, so that they will better tolerate those unfavorable environmental factors which cannot be avoided.

Fortunately there is rather abundant evidence indicating that the natural tendency in specific allergic sensitization is to lose that sensitization with the lapse of time. This is contingent in great measure upon the avoidance of repeated stimulation of the reactive mechanism by repeated exposures. Stating it more succinctly, if one will avoid an allergen long enough, one will in all probability eventually lose one's sensitization to that allergen. Thereafter, one may be exposed without resultant symptoms. The duration of necessary avoidance varies with the intensity of the sensitization. It may be short, but more often it is long, a matter of months or even years. In a series of food allergics with migraine, who found that eventually they could again eat the prohibited food without headache, the average required period of avoidance was over four years. When avoidance can be accomplished without too great inconvenience this is the preferred method.

The procedure of hyposensitization or desensitization is based upon a very early observation in the study of experimental anaphylaxis, in which it was shown that if an animal is intentionally sensitized to a foreign protein such as egg white, and is then given a second injection with an extremely small amount, not enough to cause severe reaction, the animal will thereafter tolerate even fatal doses, without symptoms. For example, let us inject 1 milligram of egg white solution into a normal guinea pig. This represents the first invasion of the enemy. After about ten days, antibodies appear in the blood, indicating that the animal has become sensitized. If, some time after this, we inject, let us say, 5 milligrams, the guinea pig will promptly die from anaphylactic shock. Let us suppose that in a series of experiments we have established that 5 milligrams is the smallest amount that will regularly kill a sensitized pig. This is then the minimal lethal dose. Now, let us take another pig sensitized in the same manner and instead of giving him a minimal lethal dose, let us give just 1 milligram, a quantity well below the fatal dose. He will have a reaction, but he will recover. After recovery, possibly the next day, let us see what the minimal lethal dose will do. We give the animal 5 milligrams, and nothing happens. He apparently remains quite well. To another treated in the same way, let us give 10 milligrams. Still nothing happens, even though this was twice the amount that should have killed the animal. These two animals are now in a state that is termed antianaphylaxis. They were allergic or anaphylactic. The injection of a very minute amount of material prior to exposing them to a large amount protected them. The antianaphylactic state does not last indefinitely. After a month or two the animals are again reactive and would again be killed with a dose of 5 milligrams.

Knowledge of the phenomenon of antianaphylaxis is the basis for the treatment of hay fever or pollinosis with pollen extracts, first successfully accomplished a little over forty years ago. It is the method employed today in desensitization against inhalant allergens. It is used at times with food allergens, bacterial vaccines and fungus extracts. It is infrequently used with drug or contact allergens. Here, avoidance or substitution is nearly always the procedure of choice.

We do not know precisely what happens in antianaphylaxis. One of the first and most generally accepted explanations was that the antibodies or defensive weapons are used up in the first or desensitizing reaction, so that nothing is left for the antigen to establish contact with when it is reintroduced. However, this doesn't fit in with our pretty little theory of the State of Allergy. Furthermore it has been demonstrated that when a person is desensitized there are just as many antibodies or reagins in the blood as there were before. Probably there are more. This fits in better with the idea that an increased number of defensive weapons are manufactured as a result of the stimulus of the attack.

Acclimatization

Or, we might explain what happens, using the analogy of acclimatization, a term which we have already employed on several occasions.

The first cold days of autumn always seem colder than do much colder days of midwinter. During the interval we have become adjusted to the lowered temperature and are not as conscious of it. In the same way the first hot days of summer cause considerable grumbling, while midsummer days of the same temperature are considered very pleasant. When one moves to the tropics, a month or two must elapse before one becomes adjusted to the new climatic conditions.

We employ this principle of acclimatization in the treatment of persons suffering from physical allergy. If such an individual experiences hives or asthma when exposed to cold, we direct him to expose himself to only a very slight degree of cold and for a short time. As soon as he finds that this no longer causes trouble the intensity and duration of the cold exposure (usually water at a specified temperature) are increased. Eventually the patient usually reaches that stage at which he can tolerate any reasonable degree of cold without experiencing symptoms.

The tissues of the person allergic to pollen or house dust are exposed to gradually increasing quantities of this allergen by means of hypodermic injections, until they reach a stage where the inhalation of previously damaging quantities produces no symptoms. Using the terminology of our story of the workers in the State of Allergy, the enemy has become naturalized. The workers find him in the community most of the time, but in such small numbers that they pay little attention to him. As the number increases, long familiarity leads to mutual readjustments so that the original antagonism no longer exists. A so-called foreign protein becomes less foreign, to the extent that the native cells are acclimated to its presence in their neighborhood. They have been able to adjust themselves so that its activity does them no damage.

Questions and Answers

Q. As I understand it, success in treatment may be achieved either by avoidance of the offending allergens or by hyposensitization. It seems to me that these two procedures are contradictory. Certainly hyposensitization, in which one is being injected repeatedly with the causative agent, would appear to be the reverse of avoidance.

A. I do not enjoy cold weather and if I can arrange to do so I shall spend my winters in the South. If this is impossible, I shall have to remain in the North, but it gets colder gradually and I will really find that in midwinter I won't mind it as much as I thought I would.

Avoidance is preferable, but if this cannot be accomplished, acclimatization by the process of hyposensitization is the alternative. Unfortunately there are many things that we cannot successfully avoid, no matter how hard we try, and we must therefore often use both methods.

There is some evidence that if hyposensitization is continued long enough, one may lose one's sensitization to the particular allergen. This has been brought out in the preceding discussion of "naturalization." The tissues gradually lose their tendency to react violently when the allergen is brought into contact with them.

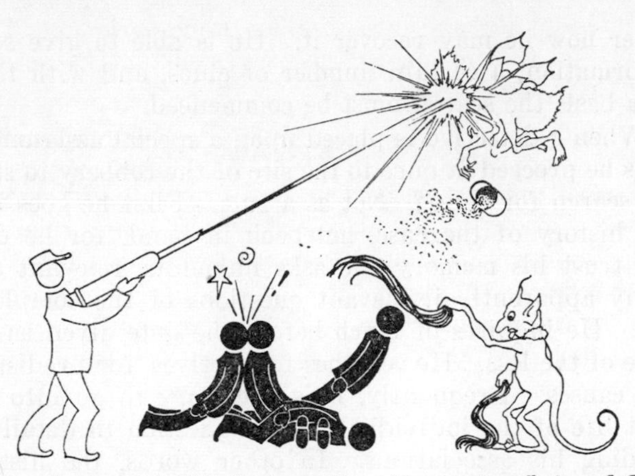

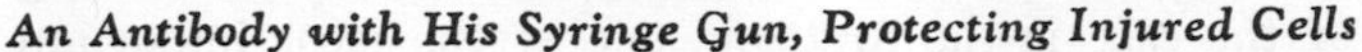

An Antibody with His Syringe Gun, Protecting Injured Cells

VII

LIAISON AND RECONNAISSANCE—TAKING INVENTORY

It is mighty difficult to fight a battle with an enemy when one doesn't even know who the enemy is. If one is being viciously attacked by an unseen or unrecognized foe, the logical procedure is to call in a detective, someone who has had experience in the procedures necessary for recognition of the trouble-maker.

Enter the doctor, with whom the patient must establish an alliance.

A Detective Game

The procedure followed by the medical consultant is very much like that used by a good detective.

The Detection of Disease

The patient presents himself to the physician with a story of having lost something. He has lost his sense of well-being, his health, and he asks that the doctor discover how he may recover it. He is able to give some information, a certain number of clues, and with these as a basis the search must be commenced.

When a detective is placed upon a special assignment, does he proceed at once to the site of the robbery to start his search for clues? Not as a rule. First he goes into the history of the case, notebook in hand, for he does not trust his memory; he asks numerous relevant and many apparently irrelevant questions of the complainant. He inquires of much before the date given as the time of the loss. He searches for motives, for predisposing causes. Frequently, it is necessary to go into the past life of the individual and to question in detail regarding his associations. In other words, the history of the case is the first and one of the most important subjects for study. This must be pursued until all possible sources of information have been exhausted.

Next, a general survey must be made. All facts are to be ascertained. All available data must be accumulated. After the complainant has told all he knows, the detective will proceed to examine the territory where the loss occurred. He will make a complete examination. He will pay as much attention to the apparently unimportant as to the apparently extremely significant phenomena. At this stage he is not stressing the important clues but is maintaining suspended judgment, noting down all facts so that later he may study them in greater detail and decide as to the relative values of each.

We are all acquainted with the story of Sherlock Holmes. Remember how Doctor Watson invariably made an incorrect diagnosis. This was because he lacked perspective and stressed unimportant bits of evidence.

Even the best detectives will overlook some clues. It is often necessary to go over the ground a second and even a third time. Frequently, special leads will turn up. These should all be followed to the end. Sometimes the detective finds a condition which he does not consider himself competent to pass upon. He may find fingerprints on a safe. He wastes little time studying these, but calls in a fingerprint expert. At times it becomes necessary to call in criminologists or other specialists.

As I have previously stated, it is extremely important that the investigator maintain a state of suspended judgment throughout the period of his inquiry. After he has acquired all available data, he will proceed to a critical analysis and will determine the important facts most intimately connected with the case. After having dissected the evidence, he will piece it together, constructing an hypothesis to explain all of the facts.

Perhaps I can better emphasize the importance of suspended judgment by the following analogy. If you were a stranger in America, unacquainted with the army uniform, and had been walking about in one of the great army camps during the war, you would have observed that all of the uniforms, both those of officers and of enlisted men, were the same. They look practically identical. Passing them hurriedly on the street, you would not notice the small metal ornament on the shoulder which alone distinguishes the general from the enlisted man. Passing them, one after another, you would be unable to decide as to relative importance. But, if later, you were to wander out onto the parade ground and there saw the troops in review you would easily recognize from the orderly arrangement of individuals into groups and of small groups into large groups that the personage of chief importance was the one riding at the head of the procession. It is only after the evidence has been sorted out by analytical methods and rearranged into coordinated groups that relative values appear.

All that I have said of the detective's routine holds equally for the methods to be followed by the diagnostician.

When the diagnostician has formulated his explanation he has not yet reached the stage of diagnosis, only that of hypothesis. It is true that, from the important clues, he has developed a possible explanation for the patient's malady. This is not the diagnosis. He may have made some error in his reasoning. Far too often medical men are content to stop at this point and to assume that the hypothesis is the final diagnosis. Much more should be done. The hypothesis must be tested and, if found to fail in the explanation of any single phenomenon or to disagree with certain observations, it must be discarded. On the basis of the discarded hypothesis a new one will then be selected. Eventually one will be developed which will fulfill all requirements and which may be designated the diagnosis.

This general program is followed by the allergist in his search for causes. The taking of a history, or, better, a discussion with the patient, is of importance greater than that of skin testing and the other diagnostic procedures. One who is adequately trained to recognize leads can often spot probable offenders in the preliminary discussion. Sensitization tests serve as a check, confirming the suspicion, or otherwise. The tests themselves are not infallible. Although they provide a wealth of important information, some of it is fallacious and may for a time lead us off on false clues. Renewed discussion with the patient after completion of the study, with a review of those substances which gave positive skin reactions or other positive tests, will often remind the patient that one or more of the positive reactors which he had completely overlooked in the first discussion actually has caused trouble in the past. This second discussion of the positive findings sometimes establishes the fact that certain of the suspected substances have been definitely proved innocuous.

It is somewhat in this manner that the physician endeavors to determine the cause of one's allergic symptoms. Knowledge of the patient's past experiences when exposed to one or another allergenic excitant, information gained from skin tests and other specific sensitization studies, and an understanding of other factors, normal and abnormal, in the patient's physical condition, general state of nutrition, his mental make-up and his customary responses to emotional stimuli, all considered in the composite picture of the problem as a whole, form the foundation upon which the physician will organize his campaign of defense or attack.

Cooperation

The physician is but a consultant, an adviser who is expert in strategy. It is the patient himself who must conduct the campaign. The doctor does not cure the patient of his allergic manifestation. With the exception of the help that he may give in desensitization he can only tell the patient what to do so that he may cure himself.

Unless the patient is willing to comply, to the letter, with the doctor's instructions he need blame no one but himself if the results are not good. Often this is no easy task. One who loves hot rolls or chocolate candy may find it difficult to resist the temptation to "take just a little," especially when his will power is being seduced by well-wishing but unintelligent friends who "can't see how just a teeny-weeny bit could possibly hurt" or by one of those less friendly foes who think that "this allergy business is all a mess of tomfoolery anyhow."

Without intelligent cooperation on the part of the patient, there will be failure on many occasions when success should have been achieved.

Questions and Answers

Q. How great a part do emotions, colds, and weather changes play in causing allergic symptoms?

A. It is only fair to say that there are a number of allergists who would not agree with the foregoing statements. They believe that allergic reactions frequently are the result of emotional disturbances alone and that people may show conditions which we consider allergic solely because of anxiety, fear, frustration and even more subtle changes in their emotional state. We have not been able to find evidence for this which we believed to be at all convincing but many excellent observers are quite convinced of its correctness.

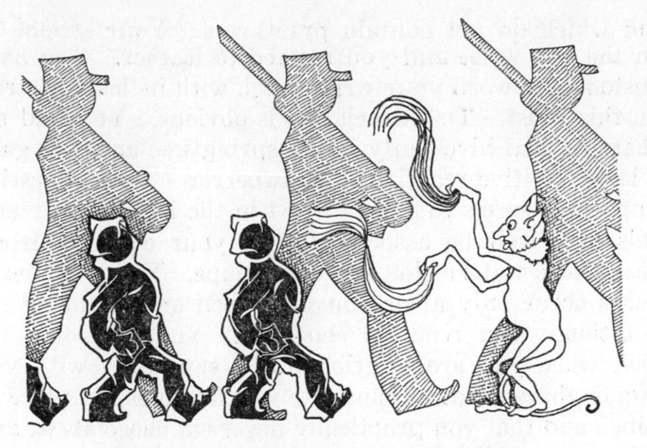

Body Cells, Protected by Antibodies

VIII

PLAN OF ATTACK—THE THERAPEUTIC PROGRAM

The doctor has completed his study. He will probably discuss the conclusions somewhat as follows.

Known Offenders

We have found that you react to this list of foods and inhalant allergens, or to such and such contact agents. Some of these fit in nicely with your own experiences. For example, you reacted to feathers and for approximately one-third of your life, eight hours of every twenty-four, you have kept your nose buried quite effectively in a feather pillow. You react to pyrethrum which is a constituent of many insect powders and sprays and you told me before we even started the study that whenever an insect spray was used in your home you promptly had asthma. If you must use insecticides, I shall give you a list of several which are easily obtained and which do not contain pyrethrum. Your eczema is on the left wrist and you reacted to leather. You have customarily worn your wrist watch with its leather strap on this wrist. The association is obvious. You told me that you had hives only in the springtime and you gave a large positive reaction to strawberries. Your digestive apparatus seems to get all upset in the late summer and this may well be associated with your equally strong reaction to watermelon and cantaloupe. Your sick headaches occur only after you have been on a hunting expedition. You react to chocolate. You have told me that when you are hunting birds, you carry with you two or three cakes of chocolate which you eat in place of lunch and that you practically never eat chocolate at any other time. Your hay fever commences around the first of March, lasting for two weeks. This is the time during which the elm trees pollinate in this climate and you have reacted positively to an extract of the elm pollen.

I shall give you instructions for the avoidance of the dust which comes from feathers in the pillows. You must also bear in mind that you cannot feed the chickens and must get rid of your canary bird and parrot. The pigeons must no longer be allowed to fly up to your bedroom window where you have been in the habit of feeding them bread crumbs. All of the foods that I have mentioned may be avoided without great inconvenience and I wish you to do this. You had better procure a metal strap for your wrist watch, preferably not of nickel since this sometimes produces sensitization and might cause trouble later on. Or you may procure one of webbed cloth, like those worn by the soldiers during the war. During the elm flowering season you will have a choice of two procedures. You might take your vacation at that time, either going to some place where elm pollination occurs at a different time, earlier or later, or where there are no elms. A trip to Bermuda or Hawaii or a West Indies cruise might do very nicely. Certainly there will be no trouble from elm pollen while you are on the ocean. The other alternative, if you find it im-

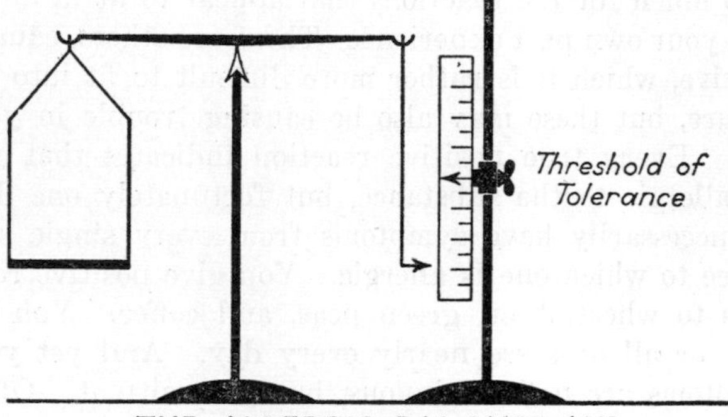

THE ALLERGIC BALANCE AND
THE YARDSTICK OF TOLERANCE

Some persons are so highly sensitized to allergens that even the smallest amount will produce symptoms. Others may tolerate small amounts but develop symptoms if exposed to larger quantities. If one who is exposed to small quantities of a specific allergen does not experience symptoms therefrom, he is in a balanced allergic state or in allergic equilibrium. He will not experience symptoms until the quantity of allergenic exposure disturbs the balance to such an extent that his threshold of tolerance is exceeded.

This and succeeding *balance* figures, from Vaughan's *Strange Malady* by permission of Doubleday, Doran & Co., Inc.

possible to get away at that time, will be desensitization. We should speak of it rather more accurately as hyposensitization, since the treatment does not completely remove the sensitization. It diminishes it sufficiently so that you are reasonably free from symptoms, but you are still sensitized.

New Possibilities

So much for the reactions that appear to fit in nicely with your own past experience. There are others, equally positive, which it is rather more difficult to fit into the picture, but these may also be causing trouble in your case. Every true positive reaction indicates that you are allergic to the substance, but fortunately one does not necessarily have symptoms from every single substance to which one is allergic. You give positive reactions to wheat, beef, green peas, and coffee. You eat some or all of these nearly every day. And yet your symptoms are not continuous, but intermittent. Often you have several successive weeks of freedom from them. The same is true of house dust, one of the things which we inhale, to which you reacted.

Even though your symptoms are intermittent, these frequent-contact allergens may be playing a part. What was said in the previous chapter about the role of emotions, colds, and weather changes in precipitating attacks is entirely applicable here. The patient may be allergic to a certain food but, as explained before, have attacks only when assisted by some accessory factor.

Changes in weather, a cold, emotional disturbance or unduc fatigue may, as nonspecific factors, precipitate attacks. Failure to recognize this fact has often led to the belief that climatic factors alone or emotional upsets may be the underlying cause of asthma or other allergic reactions. Recognition of this fact offers an explanation for why, on one occa-

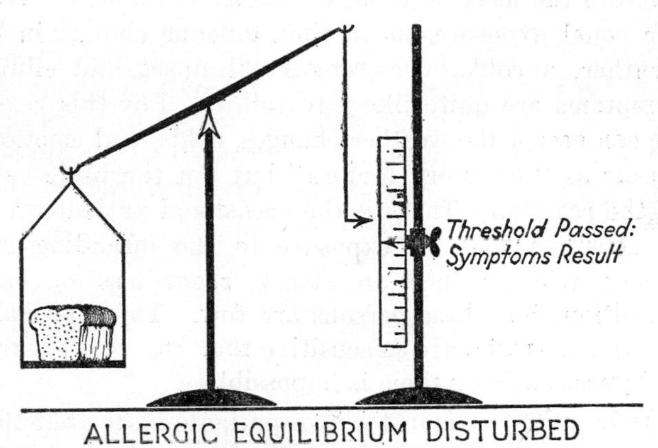

This figure illustrates how a large quantity of an allergen, such as bread, may overthrow the balance by exceeding the threshold of tolerance.

sion, the eating of some food, such as egg, may be followed by asthma while on another occasion the egg may be eaten without any asthma following. This may explain also why a patient, allergic to feathers, may sleep on a feather pillow every night but have asthma only at intervals. The explanation for this probably lies in the fact that most patients are only moderately or slightly sensitive to the antigen and, when other conditions are favorable, can tolerate the usual exposure without symptoms. Given the usual exposure and a simultaneous change in the weather, a cold, or an emotional upset and clinical symptoms are quite likely to follow. For this reason we can accept the weather changes, colds, and emotional upsets as "accessory factors" but not the basic cause of the reaction. There is the occasional patient who is so sensitive that an exposure to the offending substance will produce an attack regardless of other conditions but these persons are few. These probably are the ones who are so sensitive that any real progress in hyposensitizing them is impossible.

It is quite common to have patients state that their attacks of asthma coincide with abrupt changes in the weather or that they are much more likely to have attacks in damp weather. The hay fever patient will state that he cannot have a fan blowing on him or sit beside an open window without having his symptoms aggravated and I have seen many bald headed men who slept with skull caps, for a breeze blowing in on their bald heads would waken them with sneezing or nasal blocking. These people sneeze when they get out of bed or after a warm bath. They are quite sensitive to any chilling of the skin. This is simply the result of a vasomotor instability and is an exaggeration of a normal reaction. And, interestingly enough, these reactions all disappear when the allergic condition is

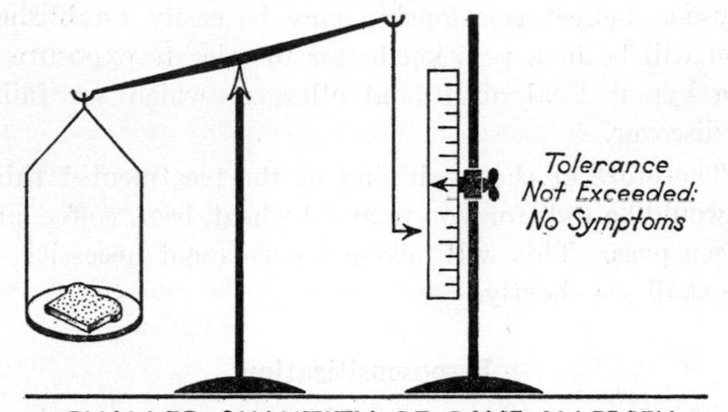
Tolerance
Not Exceeded:
No Symptoms
SMALLER QUANTITY OF SAME ALLERGEN
MIGHT BE TOLERATED

The same individual depicted in the preceding figure might tolerate a much smaller quantity of bread without exceeding his tolerance. There is an allergic reaction, as indicated by the tipping of the balance, but the reaction is not sufficiently great to produce symptoms.

controlled. A patient may state that he has asthma when the weather changes but if his allergic condition is controlled the weather may continue to change but he remains well. The same statements may be made about the influence of colds and emotional upsets.

Then there is another factor to be considered. We may not have discovered all of the allergic excitants in our first study. If you will avoid those things to which you gave positive reactions, even though no direct cause-and-effect relationship may be easily established, you will be in a position better to tolerate exposure to the hypothetical additional allergen, which we failed to discover.

Therefore at the beginning of the treatment I think it would be well for you to avoid wheat, beef, coffee, and green peas. This will not be a permanent necessity, as we shall see shortly.

Hyposensitization

Of course you cannot avoid some exposure to house dust. Possibly the lessening of the allergenic overload by the dietary restrictions just mentioned will be sufficient so that you will tolerate it in spite of continued exposure. But if you happen to have symptoms that are directly attributable to house dust, particularly respiratory symptoms, better results will be obtained, more rapidly, if we proceed to hyposensitize you with frequent injections of very small amounts of an extract of house dust. This has no dirt or germs in it. It is a chemical solution, purified and sterilized. This series of injections must be continued over a period of many months.

We can hyposensitize with practically any of the allergens which are inhaled (except chemicals) and the results are usually good. We can also hyposensitize against

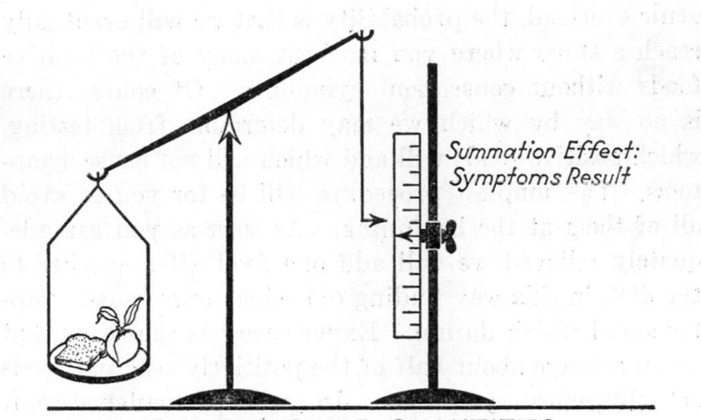

SUB-THRESHOLD QUANTITIES
OF TWO ALLERGENS MAY TOGETHER
UPSET ALLERGIC EQUILIBRIUM

A person might be allergic to these two foods and tolerate either one of them in moderation but not both together, even though they are taken in moderation.

foods and the results are frequently quite satisfactory. Contact allergens such as weeds which may produce a dermatitis are susceptible to hyposensitization.

False and Borderline Reactions

Returning now to a discussion of the foods, I have told you that not all positive reactors actually cause trouble. Although they may help to increase the allergenic overload, the probability is that we will eventually reach a stage where you may eat many of the positive foods without consequent symptoms. Of course there is no way by which we may determine from testing, which positive foods will and which will not cause symptoms. The simplest procedure will be for you to avoid all of them at the beginning. As soon as you are adequately relieved we will add one food after another to the diet, in this way finding out which ones cause symptoms and which do not. Experience has shown us that on an average about half of the positively reacting foods actually cause symptoms. In your particular case it may be that all positive reactors are responsible for trouble or it may be that only one or even none produces symptoms. Since it is easier to start out on a strictly limited diet and gradually add one food after another than it is to gradually cut away one food after another, we will start in at the hard end first. But please understand that this restricted diet is not permanent and is to be modified as you improve.

Now there are some other positive skin reactions which I have not yet mentioned. These are low-grade or borderline reactions. We have not listed these foods as "to be avoided," but when you do eat them be careful to see whether you have any symptoms which might be attributed to them. In this way you will be in a position to help us to determine whether the

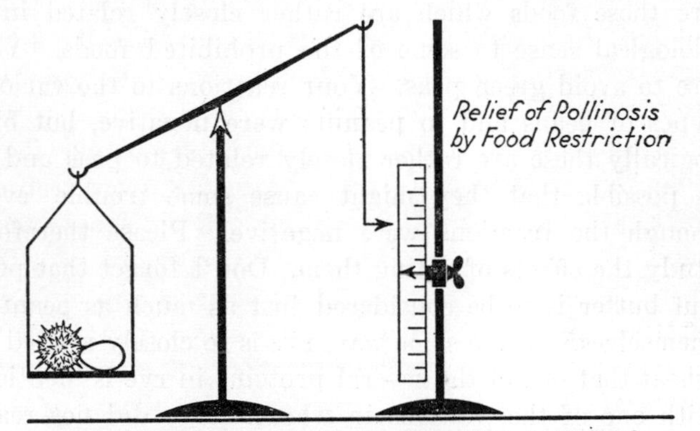

A PERSON ALLERGIC TO POLLEN AND EGG MIGHT RE-ESTABLISH TOLERANCE BY AVOIDING THE LATTER

Many persons with hay fever state that they can eat certain foods at any time of year except when they are having hay fever.

During the pollen season these foods either increase the hay fever or cause some other allergic symptoms. The above illustrates how the addition of pollen disturbs the balance, with consequent exceeding of the threshold. Conversely, a person who is mildly allergic to egg or other food, having no symptoms therefrom except in the pollen season, may improve his tolerance to pollen by avoiding egg during the pollen season.

borderline reactors are really of significance or are to be ignored.

Food Groups

There is another group of foods which we have not prohibited but which you would do well to watch. These are those foods which are rather closely related in a biological sense to some of the prohibited foods. You are to avoid green peas. Your reactions to the various types of beans and to peanuts were negative, but biologically these are rather closely related to peas and it is possible that they might cause some trouble, even though the reactions were negative. Please therefore study the effects of eating them. Don't forget that peanut butter is to be considered just as much as peanuts themselves. In the same way, rye is so closely related to wheat that one of the several proteins in rye is identical with one of the proteins in wheat. Rye did not react and you may eat pure rye bread, but if symptoms persist, try to see if there is any relationship to your eating of this bread. Rye bread as usually purchased in the bakery has some wheat flour in it and this will not do. (See page 159 for food groups.)

General Considerations

Another point is that you may feel that your symptoms are intermittent although you may actually be having some allergic response nearly all the time. Thus we have seen children whose only definite allergic complaint is intermittent attacks of asthma but who are nervous and fidgety all the time and who do not sleep well. If such a child is found also to react to, let us say, egg and milk, and if we remove these from the diet, while at the same time attending to the inhalant aller-

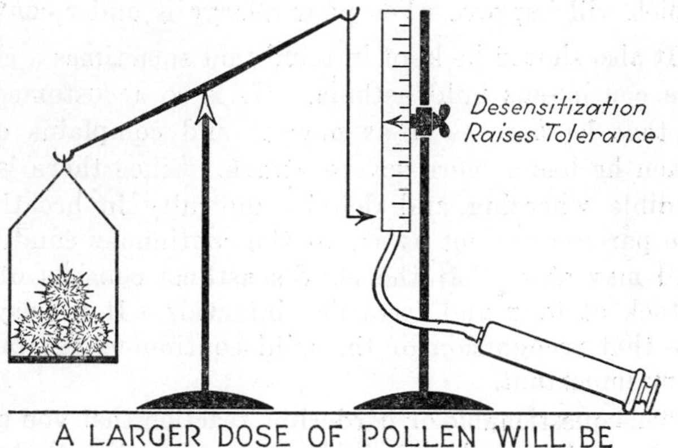
Desensitization
Raises Tolerance
A LARGER DOSE OF POLLEN WILL BE
NECESSARY TO EXCEED THRESHOLD

We may look upon desensitization or immunization against pollinosis as a process of raising the tolerance so that a larger exposure to atmospheric pollen will be required before the threshold is passed.

gens responsible for the acute asthmatic attacks, we often find that the child becomes less fidgety and sleeps better. Indefinite nervous responses of this sort may be associated with allergy. Others may do the reverse, be sleepy all the time and find relief following avoidance of daily-contact factors. Some children seem unable to gain weight satisfactorily until such factors are removed. There are many low-grade and indefinite symptoms of this sort and you may find that you have some which will improve when your allergy is under control.

It also should be kept in mind that sometimes a child has continuous mild asthma. He is so accustomed to it that he accepts it as normal and complains only when he has a more severe attack. Since there is no audible wheezing and definite difficulty in breathing the parents are not aware of the continuous condition and may state that the child's asthma consists of an attack at long and irregular intervals. It is easy to see that recognition of the mild continuous asthma is very important.

This questionable or borderline reaction that you gave to dog hair may be of significance. I realize that you have never felt that proximity to your dog caused trouble. This may be true. It may also be true that you are so fond of the dog that you don't wish to realize that he may have to go. You may have been trying to convince yourself, against your better judgment. At any rate, now that you understand the situation you will be in a position to study intelligently the results of close exposure to him.

For the present we have discussed the positive reactions, the borderline reactions, and possible biologically associated allergens, especially among the foods, which may have given false negative reactions. This brings us to a further discussion of possible false negative reactors in your particular case.

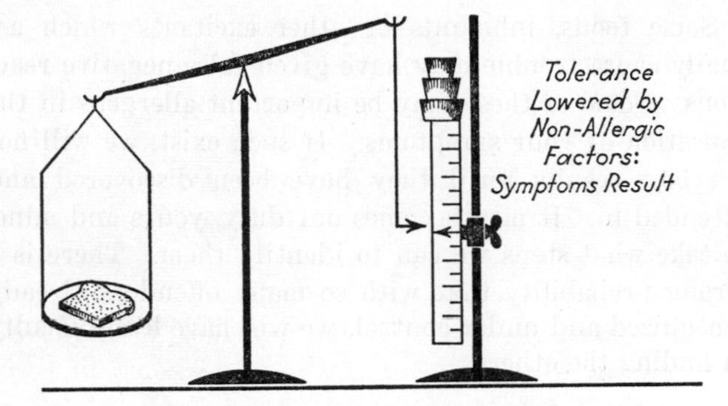

WITH INFECTION, FATIGUE, ETC.
SMALLER QUANTITIES OF ALLERGEN MAY
EXCEED THRESHOLD.

A person is allergic to bread. A large quantity exceeds his tolerance (see illustration, page 87). A small quantity, such as a single slice, does not exceed his tolerance and does not cause symptoms (see illustration, page 89). One slice may cause trouble if this person's threshold of tolerance has been lowered. Lowering may be produced by nonallergic factors, such as fatigue, excitement, worry, poisoning, constipation, bacterial infection, disturbance of the glands of internal secretion, changes in the temperature or weather or chemical factors, such as the inhalation of irritating gases, or mechanical factors as illustrated in eczema of the neck due to friction from a tight collar. Proper treatment in such cases will include not only attention to the allergenic excitants but also removal of the nonallergic factors.

Skin testing and other methods of allergic diagnostic study are not infallible. The results are not one hundred per cent accurate. Nevertheless they are the best methods available and furnish us with a truly remarkable amount of information on which we may inaugurate our campaign of attack.

Some foods, inhalants or other excitants which actually cause trouble may have given false negative reactions. Some of these may be important allergens in the causation of your symptoms. If such exist, we will not get best results until they have been discovered and attended to. It now becomes our duty, yours and mine, to take what steps we can to identify them. There is a strong probability that with so many offenders already recognized and under control, we will have less difficulty in finding the others.

The Food Diary

A very helpful method is that of keeping a diary. We will illustrate this with the food diary, although it is possible to keep a similar diary relating to contact factors and other atmospheric and environmental incidents in your daily life. The form explains in detail how to keep the food diary (see Chapter XII). Briefly, the principle is that you will record all foods eaten, all medicines taken, in fact everything that passes your lips at all times. In addition you will record your symptoms and their severity for each day. If they are due to foods and if intermittent, the diary will help us to find the offenders. You should continue the diary, if the condition is intermittent, through at least one episode and several normal days. If the condition is not intermittent after you have kept the diary for a month or longer, we will analyze it. On the summary sheet we will draw vertical red pencil lines covering those days on which you had symptoms. We will then study the foods eaten in the preceding 24 to 48 hours to see whether any certain foods were eaten only at those times. If so, they obviously come under suspicion. There are other ways in which we will analyze the diary but this is the basic principle. Of course if you are having symptoms every day there will be a red line for every day and we will be unable to get much information. But if they are mild on some days and severe on others we may be able to trace a food suspect. Furthermore, as your condition improves under the program already outlined, it is probable that although symptoms at the beginning are of daily occurrence, they will soon become intermittent. Then we will be able to get more information from the analysis. Since it will be almost as important to know what foods you were eating when you were having a lot of trouble as those eaten when symptoms are intermittent, it would be well to keep the diary irrespective of the degree of improvement.

Experience has shown us that as a rule no single food stands out in the diary as clearly responsible for exacerbation of symptoms. More often there are several *possible* offenders. You can readily see that this method will not tell us positively that this or that food is responsible. The best that we can derive from it will be that such and such foods look suspicious. Thereafter it will be up to you to watch them, studying the effects of their repeated ingestion. Or, when we reach that stage at which several foods are under suspicion you can return to the office for further study at which time we will conduct special tests, just with these foods, tests which may be positive although the original ones were negative.

The Elimination Diet

If symptoms, presumably due to foods, persist and are of too frequent occurrence for the food diary to be helpful, we shall have to approach the problem from a slightly different angle. We shall then try what is called the elimination diet, or the trial diet. This will be a very restricted diet, limited to not more than six or eight foods, those to which we have found that you react negatively by all the tests that have been applied, and foods which from experience we have found to be rather infrequent causes of allergic sensitization among people generally. If you should be relieved on this diet, then we will gradually add one food after another, thus discovering those which will cause symptoms, and establishing those which will not. The simplest elimination diet would consist of nothing but milk. This contains so many of the food elements that one can exist on it alone for days or a week or two, long enough for us to determine whether the avoidance of all other foods will relieve symptoms. Of course if you have already been found allergic to milk this will not do, and a special selection of foods as mentioned above will be made.

Only the Beginning

You can readily see from the foregoing discussion that the program as outlined is a preliminary one which without doubt will require modification from time to time, depending upon how you improve. From the nature of the allergic diseases it is usually impossible to select the perfect final program at this stage of the investigation. Although we have completed the allergic diagnostic study we have only commenced, in a sense, and the final result will depend in great measure upon the efficiency with which you and I continue our collaboration from now on.

Questions and Answers

Q. You have talked about the Food Diary and mentioned the possibility of other types of diaries. How can similar programs be applied in inhalant allergy, asthma and hay fever, which are the complaints in such a large proportion of allergics?

A. Not only is an asthmatic whose asthma is primarily due to an inhalant allergen usually also sensitized to some food, but such a person as a rule has some more or less minor allergic symptom, besides his asthma, which may be attributed to food allergy. Furthermore, an allergenic food may be responsible for at least a portion of the asthmatic episodes. Therefore, inhalant allergics should also be tested for food allergy. This holds for adults as well as children although children are rather more likely to experience asthma due to foods.

If a person with inhalant allergy is placed on a presumably nonallergenic die and symptoms persist in spite of the application of the food diary and elimination or trial diets, then it becomes probable that other factors, particularly inhalant factors, are playing the dominant part. Further study in this direction is quite analogous to the study with the food diary and elimination diets.

The inhalant diary would contain notations such as the following: Went to the stable; rode horseback; went hunting; made up the beds; house cleaning; cooked dinner; tried a new face powder; went to the hairdresser; was at a bridge party where everyone was smoking; brought down some clothes from the attic; mowed the lawn; spent the day in the country; the flowers in the living room are wilting; went to an air-conditioned "movie"; cleaned the kennel; spent some time down cellar. All such observations may be of significance to the physician. When he analyzes the diary he will have occasion to add other possible factors such as the pollen or fungus spore prevalences in the air from day to day. He will have determined these each day by actual air analysis.

The analogue to the elimination diet consists in placing the patient in a special allergen proof room, usually in a hospital, from which, by various procedures and substitutions, all known inhalant and contact allergic excitants are barred at all times.

Q. You speak of related foods as causing symptoms, even though some members of the group are positive and others negative. Do these related foods always cause trouble?

A. The specificity of sensitization may be limited to a certain food or other substance or it may include several closely related substances. Thus one person may be allergic to peanut without being sensitized to peas or beans; while a second reacts to peas and beans, but not to peanuts; a third to peas and peanuts but not to beans; and a fourth to all three.

When one is sensitized to only a single substance in a biologic group we speak of it as species specificity. When he reacts to all the members of a group we speak of it as family or group specificity.

Q. Does this apply only to foods or may it apply to other allergens?

A. This may apply to any closely related substances. Thus some persons are allergic only to goose feathers while others react to feathers from all sources. The first is an example of species sensitization, the latter an example of group specificity. There are similar crossed reactions between the hair or dander of horse, zebra, and donkey.

The same holds with the pollens. There are a number of grass pollens which may cause hay fever. Some persons react to all or nearly all of them, while others do so only to one or two of the members of the grass family.

Q. If one reacts to hen's egg may one eat chicken?

A. Occasionally a person is found to react to chicken feathers, chicken meat, and hen's egg. This is unusual.

More often there is no definite correlation between these three allergens. Of course they all contain chicken protein, but there are several different types of protein in chicken as in all other animals and one may be sensitized to one of these proteins derived from one part of the animal and not to others derived from different parts. A person who is allergic to horse serum may or may not have trouble from inhaling horse dander.

Q. If one is highly sensitized to corn isn't it possible that this person would react to the flesh of an animal or fowl whose diet had been largely corn?

A. It has been shown that allergens eaten by the animal may, after absorption through the intestinal tract and into the blood, pass into the milk and be delivered to the ultimate consumer in this manner. Thus, egg allergen has been shown to be present in mother's milk. There is evidence that a person who is allergic to cottonseed may have trouble from drinking cow's milk if the cow has been fed cottonseed meal.

There is no definite evidence that one who is allergic to corn or peanuts will experience an allergic reaction after eating ham from a corn-fed or peanut-fed hog.

Q. After I am adequately relieved, how rapidly may I add foods back into the diet in order to determine which ones actually are responsible for symptoms?

A. One of the difficulties of food sensitization is that an allergic food need not necessarily produce symptoms every time it is eaten. It may cause trouble at one time, and not at another. A person might "get away with it" when eating the food occasionally, but find himself in trouble after eating it several days in succession.

It does not suffice, therefore, to add a new food every day. Each food being tried should be taken for from three to four successive days before one may safely conclude that it is innocuous, and proceed with trial of the next food. During these days a generous amount of the food should be eaten each day—as much as you are likely to eat in any day—so that, if you are ever to react to this food, you will do it now.

A food which causes symptoms during trial must be avoided.

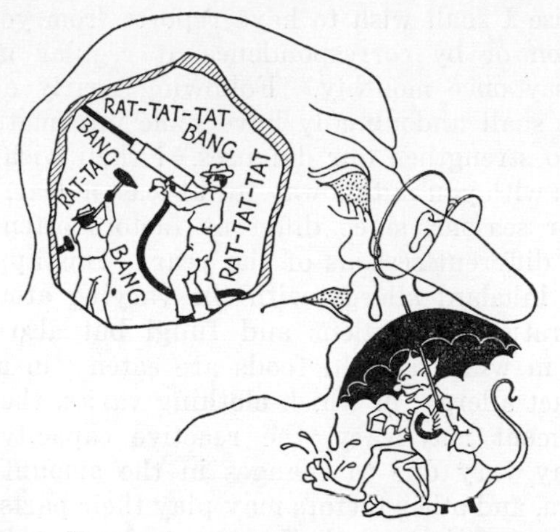

Allergic Headache, Hay Fever, and Conjunctivitis

IX

A WAR OF ATTRITION— THE LONG DRAG

The doctor will probably continue with his monologue somewhat as follows:

If we are eventually to come out victorious in our future battles with the allied forces of the enemy, you and I will have to cooperate in nearly every step of the campaign. We might look upon yourself as the advance guard, busy with reconnaissance, continually engaged, while protecting yourself, in efforts to gain new information concerning the identity, location, and strength of the enemy and sending these reports back to me, stationed far behind the lines at G. H. Q. and attempting to coordinate the defense, by remote control.

"Military Intelligence"

If you are to receive hyposensitizing therapy I shall be seeing you at regular intervals for this purpose.

Otherwise I shall wish to have reports from you either in person or by correspondence at regular intervals, let us say once monthly. Following nearly every report we shall undoubtedly have some information with which to strengthen our defenses. I shall wish to keep in touch with you in this way for at least a year, through the four seasons, since different factors often play a part at different seasons of the year. This applies not only to inhalant allergy with the varying atmospheric concentrations of pollens and fungi but also to food allergy in which certain foods are eaten "in season"; to contact allergy, in which clothing varies, the general environment may vary, the reactive capacity of the skin may vary due to changes in the amount of perspiration, and other factors may play their parts. Plants such as poison ivy, weeds, grasses, and trees which may cause contact dermatitis are "in season." Finally the excitants of physical allergy, heat, cold, and sunlight vary with the seasons. During the first year some or all of these factors will be taken into consideration for any future modification of your therapeutic program.

There are many things concerning which you will be making records. Of those mentioned in the preceding discussion, you will be reporting concerning the possible relief of such indefinite symptoms as insomnia and nervousness, sleepiness, general fatigue, various indefinite neuritic types of pain, constipation, diarrhea, low-grade digestive upsets, which you may find improved. You will be reporting concerning your response to borderline reactors and to negatively reacting foods biologically related to positive foods. Since you will be on the lookout for possible new factors, you may be reporting concerning hitherto unsuspected substances which you think might be playing a part. Since you will be studying your food diary on your own initiative, you may be able to discover certain false-negative foods, yourself, and will undoubtedly mention some that you suspect when you send in your food diary. Possibly you will develop similar ideas from the inhalant or the contact diary.

Nonspecific Measures

There is another phase of your treatment which I have not previously mentioned and which may turn out to have some importance in future analysis of the progress of your case. Until now we have discussed only the specific allergic treatment. One might infer that prior to the development of this modern method there was no treatment whatsoever available for asthma, hay fever, migraine, eczema, hives, gastrointestinal symptoms due to food idiosyncrasy or for the more obscure allergic manifestations. As a matter of fact many sufferers were treated with reasonable success by methods which we might designate as nonspecific, in contradistinction to the specificity of the allergic procedures. Nonspecific measures included such as the treatment of focal infection in the teeth, tonsils, sinuses or elsewhere; relief of constipation; the prescribing of glasses in the case of migraine; soothing ointments in eczema; treatment of disorders of the glands of internal secretion such as the thyroid, pituitary and ovaries; protection against fatigue and especially against various causes of abnormal emotional upsets; and above all, improvement in the patient's general constitution, his nutrition, his muscular tone, his over-all state of well-being. These general nonspecific measures are as important for ultimate best results today as they have been in the past. For this reason I shall give you special instructions concerning those factors which are of significance in your own case.

I have told you how two allergens may act in a cumulative way and how the removal of one tends to increase tolerance toward the others. Nonspecific agents such as those listed above may act in a similar way as predisposing factors. A person reactive to wheat may have symptoms only when he becomes fatigued or has a cold. Control of these nonspecific factors will often increase tolerance to the specific ones (see illustration on page 97).

Therefore, in your diary, you will also wish to report episodes of this sort and intercurrent illnesses such as a toothache, an ordinary head cold, and the like.

Avoidance of Nonessentials

At this stage we are likely to encounter yet another difficulty. I have told you of so many things that should be included in your various diaries and in your monthly reports that you may be afraid to leave anything out of your reports, lest it be of importance. As a consequence the report will be so cluttered up with nonessentials that it will be quite impossible for the doctor to separate the wheat from the chaff. You now have a nice little problem in judgment as to what should be included and what should not. And since you are the only person who is with yourself all day, you are the one best qualified to judge as to what should go into the report. If, however, your doctor tells you that you have given him too much detail, suggesting that in the future you omit this and that item, don't be offended. You and he are both working toward the same end and his suggestion is made so that you can both reach it sooner.

The Need for Adequate Nutrition

Before we leave the subject of diet one other point should be mentioned. The food which you will be eating during the period of continued investigation will probably be restricted in variety. As additional foods come under suspicion there may be still further restrictions. It is important that the doctor see to it that your nourishment is ample for your needs, that you have sufficient protein, fats, carbohydrates, minerals, and especially vitamins. This does not usually become such a problem that foods must be weighed or measured, and calories counted. As a rule, the various nutritional elements may be obtained from a selection of such a wide variety of foods that one need have no worries concerning dietary deficiencies. However if this does become a problem it will be the duty of the doctor to so rearrange the diet as to prevent deficiencies. If the diet cannot be arranged to provide a sufficiency of the needed vitamins, many of these are fortunately now prepared synthetically or in concentrates and may be taken in tablet or liquid form, just like medicines.

Rapid Relief

I presume that I have given the impression that in every case it is a long drag, a matter of months or years before relief is obtained. This is not true. In the large majority of cases the important offenders are all found on the first diagnostic study and improvement thereafter is rapid. It is not unusual to observe fully 75 per cent relief within two or three weeks after the inauguration of treatment, sometimes sooner. The last 25 per cent is likely to be much slower, and will depend principally upon constant adherence to the program as outlined and as modified from time to time. In the case of hay fever, when treatment is commenced during the season, some relief is usually obtained within five to seven days, sometimes indeed within a few hours after the first hyposensitizing injection. Results with pollen asthma may be as rapid although they are more often somewhat slower.

The point which I wish to emphasize is that if relief does not occur promptly you should not become discouraged. Sensitization is usually multiple. If there are, let us say, twelve substances to which you are allergic and only nine or ten of them are found at the preliminary study, you will not obtain best results until the additional two or three are identified. This often requires considerable time. Not infrequently it calls for most painstaking cooperation between doctor and patient. So, if after a month or two or three you are no better, don't conclude that the doctor is all wrong, and give up, but cooperate to the best of your ability, helping him to help you. There may be several occasions when you will have every reason to be discouraged, when your attacks are just as bad as they ever were and possibly just as frequent, but bear in mind that it is sometimes a long drag, and keep on trying.

The results of perseverance are well illustrated in a series of cases with allergic headache. In this disease especially, nonspecific factors are likely to play an important role, causing a relatively high proportion of the attacks. These tend to obscure the allergic causes and on many occasions have caused the doctor as well as the patient to give up. The particular series mentioned was divided into two groups, those who were ultimately relieved and those who were not. The former collaborated with the allergist for an average period of eighteen months, the latter for but six. Presumably the second group became discouraged too soon although we are not justified in claiming that if they had continued for eighteen months they would have done better. They may have been the more severe cases or they may have been those in whom the allergic factor was of less importance than the nonspecific factors. The fact remains, however, that treatment must sometimes be persisted in for a long time.

Slow Improvement

This is well illustrated in the cases described in Charts I and II. Mr. A. charted weekly summaries of the severity and duration of his respiratory symptoms. He consulted an allergist at the point indicated by the first arrow (August). Treatment was instituted and in the ensuing month his symptoms were much improved. He next saw the allergist at the point indicated by the second arrow. In the months just preceding, his symptoms had again become aggravated, it appeared that the treatment had failed, and he had every reason for his discouragement. However, analysis of the chart brought out a previously unsuspected finding, that there was evidence of a seasonal variation. The prediction was made

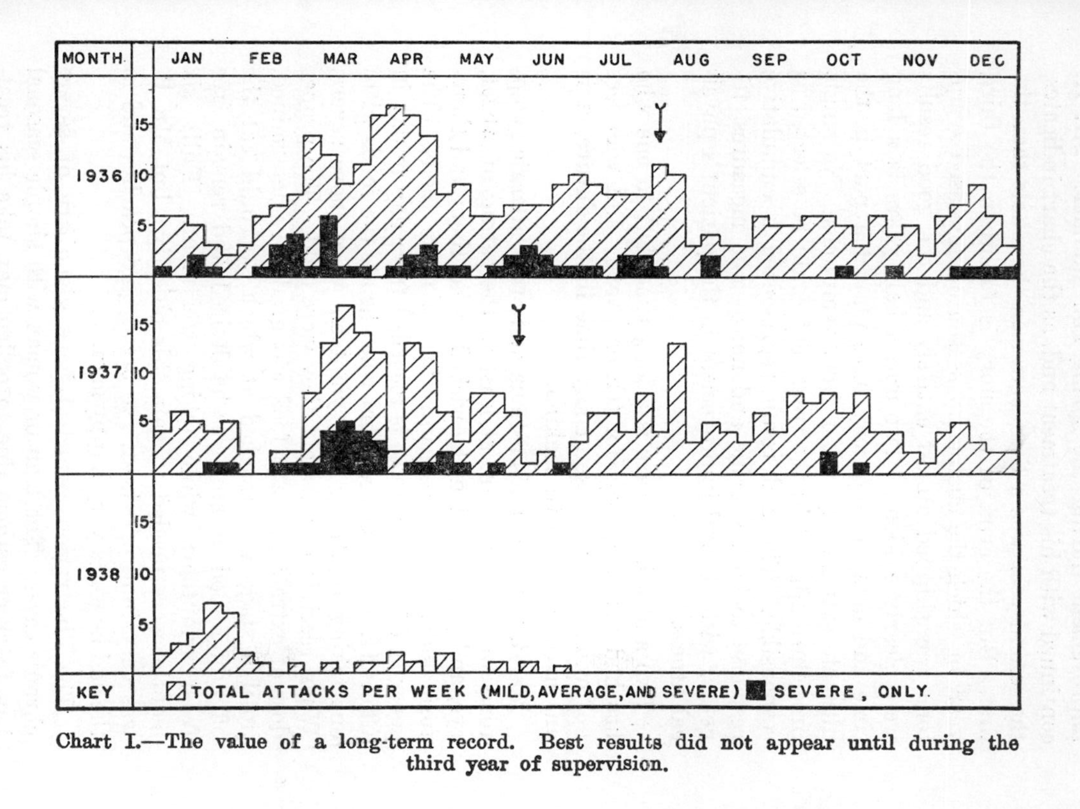

Chart I.—The value of a long-term record. Best results did not appear until during the third year of supervision.

that with this season passed, there would be still greater improvement during the spring and summer. Mr. A. continued with his treatment and, as the chart indicates, the second year was a little better on the whole than the first. But the crux of the story is found in the third year, in which the customary season of increased symptoms was skipped almost entirely and the good results were clearly evident. Two and a half years is a long time and many things may have played a part in the ultimate satisfactory relief from symptoms. No single procedure applied in the treatment could be selected as responsible. The end result represented a cumulative response to both specific and nonspecific measures, together with general improvement in the patient's physical fitness.

Two and a half years is a long time, but to one who has had his symptoms for ten or twenty and who sees no promise of surcease at any time in the future, it is an investment worth making.

Mr. B. knew that his asthma and other allergic symptoms were due in part at least to the eating of wheat, rye, and peaches. But he wished to eat them and therefore undertook hyposensitization to these foods. The severity of his symptoms is recorded from day to day in Chart II. It will be seen that when he ate the foods without taking treatment his symptoms were more severe. When receiving treatment they were mild. The proper dose of extract for each food was gradually determined, until a stage was reached at which he could eat the offending food as much as he desired and remain free from symptoms, while taking treatment. Fully six months were needed to gain this objective, but Mr. B. was very fond of wheat, rye bread, and peaches and in the end he was a very happy man.

The illustrations which I have given are of severe chronic cases. The man or woman with simple seasonal hay fever or asthma due to pollen may take his treatment prior to the season or throughout the year, remain-

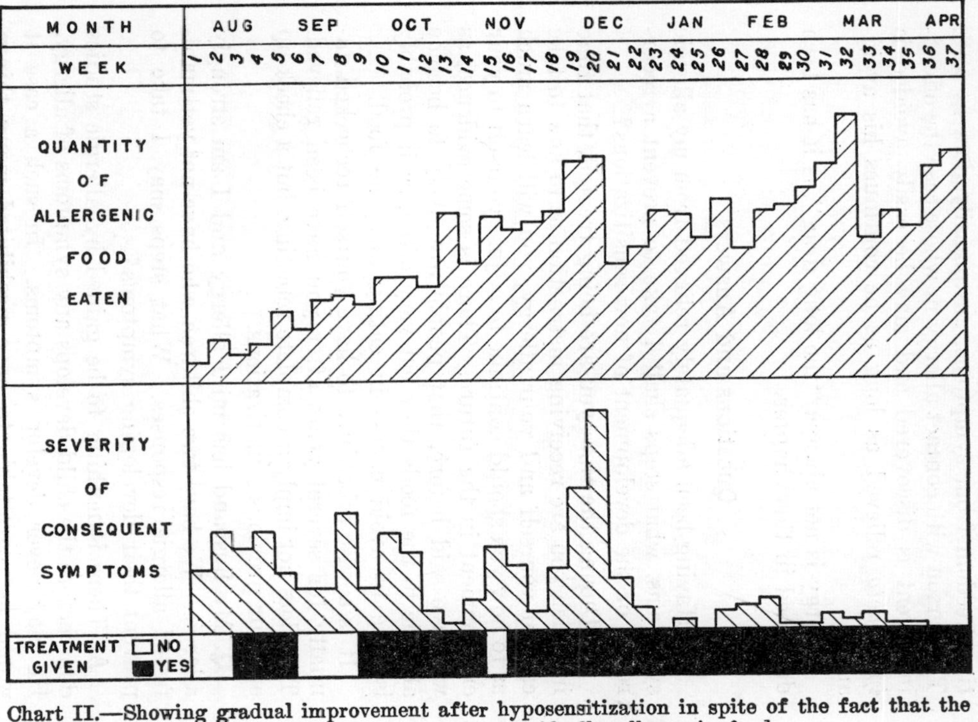

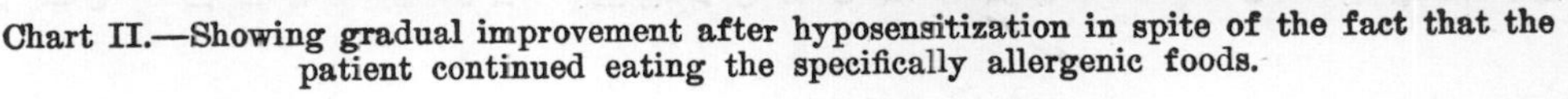

Chart II.—Showing gradual improvement after hyposensitization in spite of the fact that the patient continued eating the specifically allergenic foods.

ing symptom-free or nearly so at all times. The person with seasonal symptoms or acute allergic episodes occurring at intervals, with intervening periods of entire freedom from symptoms, customarily does as well. The person with contact allergy in whose case the offending agent is discovered and may be easily avoided is *ipso facto* relieved as long as he continues his avoidance.

Allergy is not always "the long drag" as it has been described in this chapter.

Questions and Answers

Q. Having been adequately relieved from my allergic symptoms, what steps shall I take to prevent a recurrence, or the development of new sensitizations?

A. During the time you are being treated, that time in which you are receiving instruction as to how to take care of yourself and your allergy, you will learn much as to how you should continue to adjust yourself to your environment in the future. There is some evidence, as we have said before, that people are likely to become allergic to the foods they eat very often, so it probably is wise to avoid excess in eating any one food.

It is a wise procedure to have yourself rechecked annually for several years after you have been relieved. This does not imply a complete retesting, but a check-up on your previous sensitizations.

Q. My husband has mild allergy and I am strongly allergic. We have two children who have not yet manifested allergic responses. What steps may I take to prevent their developing symptoms?

A. There is nothing to be gained by allergic studies done before the child develops any symptoms of allergy. He may never develop symptoms. In such a case it would be regrettable to have prohibited many things unnecessarily.

The important point to remember is that if allergic symptoms do develop, no matter how mild they may be, then you should have an allergic study made without delay. The earlier the abnormal reaction is adjusted the more rapidly will the patient recover. It is much easier to control one or a few sensitizations than it is later to adjust the person who reacts to a large number of substances.

The larger the number of sensitizations which an individual has, the more the likelihood of his developing additional ones. A person who continues exposure to his allergen, with resulting symptoms, is more likely to develop new sensitizations. These two statements have not been proved, but there is considerable clinical evidence indicating their probable truth. If they are true, they indicate the need for early recognition of the causes, and appropriate treatment.

Aside from this, about all that you can do with your allergically predisposed children will be to keep them in the best possible general health and to have them avoid dietary indiscretions and other types of excesses. But don't carry your solicitude too far. Children are often splendid imitators. If taught to anticipate the development of symptoms "just like mother's or father's," they may, quite unconsciously, evolve complaints which are primarily psychogenic in origin.

Q. You mentioned asthma, hay fever, sick headaches, eczema, angioneurotic edema, hives, and some forms of indigestion as the allergic diseases. Are there others?

A. These are the common allergic diseases. There are several others in which allergy appears to play a part. Serum sickness (hives and other symptoms occurring after an injection of therapeutic serum) is allergic and was the first disease recognized as such. Agranulocytosis, also called malignant neutropenia, agranulocytic angina, and granulopenia, is a very serious condition, fortunately uncommon, in which sensitization to certain drugs appears to be a causative factor. Certain forms of purpura or abnormal bleeding have been found associated with food or drug allergy. There is an unusual disease of the blood vessels known as periarteritis nodosa, believed to be allergic. Ivy poisoning is a manifestation of contact allergy.

Allergic headache need not necessarily be migrainous or "sick headache" in type. Occasionally, neuritis, transient paralysis, and unexplained chronic fatigue are allergic. So also are several types of eye disease.

Other diseases in which there is some evidence of an allergic factor, at times at least, include recurrent canker sores, cyclic vomiting, pylorospasm, mucous colitis, Ménière's disease, erythema multiforme, and thromboangiitis obliterans. Regarding some of these, more conclusive evidence is needed before we can say definitely concerning their allergic causation.

Also there are conditions which sometimes are allergic and at other times are not. For example, some headaches are undoubtedly allergic while certainly most headaches are not. We have seen episodes closely resembling appendicitis or gall bladder disease which were due to allergy. We have seen hemorrhage from the bowel due to drugs but it remains true that most hemorrhage from the bowel is not allergic. Allergy can be a great imitator of organic disease and often has to be carefully differentiated from some organic condition.

X

THE MINUTE MEN IN THE FRONT LINE

If we wish to continue the analogy of the body's defenses to the military forces, we may liken the medication we use to the minute men, the local guard, who can be mobilized immediately, go into combat at once, and whose function is to control the situation until other forces can be brought up. For medicines used in the treatment of allergic conditions are for prompt relief. They do not cure. They are very important as a means of controlling conditions which, though seldom fatal, are none the less alarming and disabling. We need specific treatment to keep allergic persons well, but when an episode occurs, such as an attack of asthma, a violent bout of hay fever, or a disabling urticaria, it is important to be able to give prompt and satisfactory relief.

The purpose of this chapter is not to teach you so much about the medicines used in allergy that you may carry on your own medication. That is always a dangerous thing to attempt. Chiefly, it is written with the hope that we may give you a bird's eye view of what the doctor is trying to do when he gives you these medicines and also to correct a number of misapprehensions that many people have about these drugs.

Fifty years ago there was little that could be done for the asthmatic patient. Salts of iodine were used in patent medicines as well as in doctors' prescriptions. Sometimes they helped a great deal. Arsenic was used in some prescriptions and is still used by some physicians, but it is a dangerous drug to use over a long period of time because of the danger of arsenic poisoning, so it is seldom used. A nasal spray for the relief of hay fever and asthma which used to be quite popular depended upon cocaine for its effectiveness, and this, of course, was always a dangerous procedure.

About fifty years ago Takamine, a chemist, succeeded in extracting EPINEPHRINE from the adrenal gland and it was given the trade name of ADRENALIN. It was found that this substance given hypodermically was a very excellent drug for the relief of the asthmatic paroxysm. It still remains the most valuable drug we have for this purpose. Its action is rapid but brief and it may have to be repeated at intervals. Its action is too short for it to be of much help in urticaria or eczema. Many people have failed to take advantage of the great help which may be had from the use of this drug because they have been told that it is very likely to injure the heart. This is not correct. It may be used, when used properly, in repeated doses without doing any damage whatever and it is by far the best single control measure we have. Children require epinephrine in much the same dosage as adults and take it as safely.

There are a number of sprays on the market which are satisfactory in the relief of asthma which is not very severe. They are sold under different names but all are forms of epinephrine. They can be helpful particularly in that they can always be available and used promptly day or night, but they should be used with discretion and following the directions of a physician.

Epinephrine may cause a tremor and a pallor of the skin. It may cause the heart to "pound" briefly and may raise the blood pressure slightly. None of these symptoms is important enough to preclude the use of the drug. Because of fear many patients postpone taking epinephrine until it becomes quite obvious that something must be done. This is a mistake. If there ever was a place where "A stitch in time saves nine," it is here. Treatment for the relief of an asthmatic attack should be started as soon as it appears that an attack is developing. A small amount of medication then may be much more effective than a lot more taken later. When using treatment for relief of asthma, "Do it now."

EPHEDRINE is a drug used by the Chinese for many years and for many purposes. When it was found to be a helpful drug for the relief of asthma and hay fever it immediately became popular and was used widely. A great advantage over epinephrine is that it can be used orally and also that its action is more prolonged. A disadvantage is that it causes a great many people to become quite nervous and wakeful. For this reason it is usually combined with small amounts of a sedative.

Several other drugs, chemically much like ephedrine or epinephrine, and with much the same therapeutic action, have been made. Neo-Synephrine and Propadrine are two of these that serve as examples. These do not produce the nervousness caused by ephedrine but neither are they quite as effective.

Ephedrine and its "analogues" are used orally and sometimes hypodermically for the relief of asthma but chiefly their greatest usefulness is found in the treatment of hay fever or urticaria. In hay fever they are often used as a spray or drops in the nose. They also may be used in the eye for relief of irritation in hay fever or allergic conjunctivitis.

AMINOPHYLLIN and THEOPHYLLIN have proved to be quite helpful to the asthmatic person. They frequently give relief for several hours and, given intravenously, may give relief when epinephrine has failed. They can be given orally but relieve only the mild attacks. Used in the form of a rectal suppository they may be almost as effective as in an intravenous injection. It is possible now to cover a tablet with such a coating that it requires approximately four hours to dissolve it, consequently the patient begins to get the effect of the drug about four hours after taking it. This can be very helpful in the patient who goes to bed and to sleep but awakes at two or three o'clock in the morning with asthma. A coated tablet of aminophyllin taken at bed time may make it possible for such a patient to sleep through the night without interruption.

Aminophyllin and theophyllin frequently cause nausea sufficient to interfere with their use.

Everyone has heard of, and many people have used, one of the ANTIHISTAMINIC DRUGS which came on the market a few years ago. There are now thirty or more of them, all used for the same purpose and believed to act in the same way. Their purpose is to nullify the action of histamine which is assumed to be the cause of the allergic reaction.

Some of these drugs are more effective than others, the action of some is more prolonged, and some of them do not produce unpleasant effects as often as do others. The very interesting and peculiar fact about these drugs is that there is no "best drug." One may be quite effective with some people and relatively ineffective with others. The one which gives you a great deal of help may not help your neighbor at all.

The same statement may be made relative to the unpleasant effects of these drugs. One of them may produce drowsiness, nervousness, nausea, and many other effects in more patients than does another, but the one which often produces trouble in others may not cause any in you.

There is no way to determine which of these drugs will be most helpful with the least unpleasantness, except to try them and see. If you find one which appears sufficiently potent and has no unpleasant effects, use it.

Another defect of these drugs is that after continued use—sometimes for a short time, sometimes much longer—relief may suddenly stop. When this happens you may be able to find another drug which will be helpful, for a while.

These are not the wonder-working drugs they were first thought to be. In addition to the defects just mentioned, we should state that they are of little or no help in the treatment of asthma. Also, in the treatment of hay fever, we find that, when the pollen count is low, the drugs seem quite helpful, but, when the count is high, the patient has hay fever in spite of the medication.

These drugs may be used orally, as a nasal spray, intravenously, and in an ointment. They may help to control hay fever symptoms particularly when used in conjunction with pollen therapy. In an ointment they may give relief from much of the itching of allergic eczema but they have little or no beneficial effect upon the eruption itself. These drugs used on the skin seem to be good "sensitizers" and may themselves aggravate the eruption, so they must be watched carefully.

The ANTIBIOTICS, particularly PENICILLIN, have been used a great deal in the treatment of asthma. They are helpful in asthma complicated by respiratory infection and are much used in those cases in which the asthma is believed due to a bacterial infection. They are of no help at all in the noninfected cases although, we regret to say, they have been used quite indiscriminately. These drugs may be used by mouth, hypodermically, or by inhalation.

The term "miracle drug" has been applied to many medicaments but to none more frequently than to ACTH, CORTISONE and HYDROCORTISONE. ACTH (which is a simple way of saying adreno-corticotropic hormone) is a substance formed by the pituitary gland. This substance then acts upon the adrenal gland which, in turn, produces cortisone, hydrocortisone, and other "steroid" substances. ACTH and cortisone have been found to give remarkable relief in a number of conditions, including the allergic manifestations. How they produce these results is not known. Unfortunately, the effect is only temporary and when the treatment is stopped the symptoms recur. The exceptions to this statement are the self-limited conditions such as poison ivy dermatitis or a contact dermatitis the cause of which can be avoided. For an asthmatic attack which has got out of control by the usual medication, these agents can be extremely helpful. They can bring about relief of severe attacks in a short time and may be invaluable in these cases. Careful supervision by the physician is necessary since some bad effects may develop unless prevented by suitable action. There are also some conditions in which the use of these drugs is definitely contraindicated. Diseases such as tuberculosis, peptic ulcer, nephritis, etc., may be made very much worse by the use of these drugs.

ACTH is used hypodermically or intravenously while cortisone and hydrocortisone can be used in tablet form orally, or for local use in solution or ointment.

These substances are of great value and can be very helpful in selected cases but their limitations are definite and contraindications are certain. They are not cures but are unexcelled for getting patients "over a bad hump." And the knowledge that has been gained with these agents may help in the discovery of other knowledge which may lead to still more effective control of allergic conditions.

One form of treatment needs to be mentioned only to be condemned. This is the use of OPIATES in the treatment of the asthmatic paroxysm. This is dangerous practice and deaths have resulted from it. With the agents we now have available there is no necessity for the use of opiates, and they should be scrupulously avoided.

The foregoing discussion does not mention all the drugs which may be employed in the treatment of allergic conditions. They are many, but those discussed are the important ones and serve to show what can be done with medicinal agents in the control of allergy. We have talked about them so that you may know a little about them and understand what the doctor is trying to accomplish when he uses them.

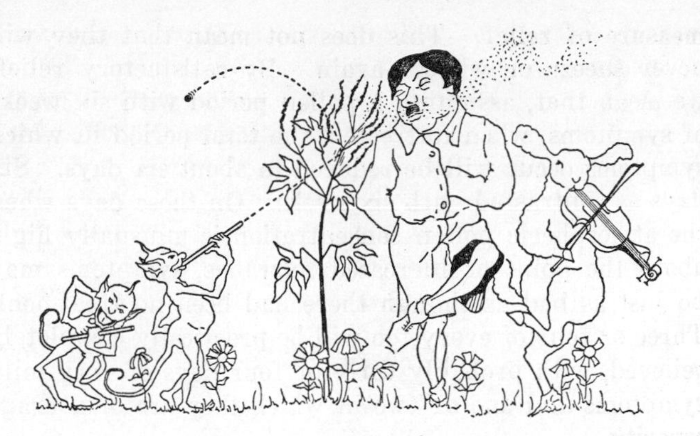

The Dance of the Seasons

XI

VICTORY OR DEFEAT?

What is the usual outcome of allergic therapy? Is the defensive war, waged in the manner described in preceding chapters, usually successful, or does one continue to suffer? If I take an entire chapter to answer this question, as I fully intend to do, you will have every justification for anticipating all sorts of hedging and evading of the question and the insertion of a large number of *ifs* and *buts* and *ands* and *althoughs*, as necessary stage equipment to make the story have a happy ending. This is not the case. A straightforward answer may be given in a few words and you will find these in the next paragraphs. In an effort to point out some of the obstacles to recovery and the best methods of avoiding them, the remainder of the chapter is devoted primarily to those who fail at first to achieve the relief which they have been led to anticipate.

Results of Treatment

Eight or nine out of every ten persons with seasonal hay fever, properly treated, will obtain a satisfactory measure of relief. This does not mean that they will never sneeze or wheeze again. By satisfactory relief, we mean that, assuming a pollen period with six weeks of symptoms, when untreated, the total period in which symptoms occur will be reduced to about six days. Six days as contrasted with six weeks. On those days when the atmospheric pollen concentration is unusually high, above the point of increased tolerance, symptoms may be just as bad as though there had been no treatment. Three or four of every ten will be practically completely relieved, with probably three or four days of very mild symptoms and one or two in which they are of average severity.

Patients with asthma and hay fever occurring throughout the year, either quite steadily or at frequent intervals, with no clear-cut seasonal variation, must be divided into two groups. The first group, in whom study demonstrates that the offending allergen comes from outside of the body (so-called "extrinsic" cases) will find that about seven or eight of each ten receive altogether satisfactory relief. The second group comprises those who cannot be shown to react to skin testing nor proved to be sensitive by other methods. These persons are usually past middle life and develop their allergic condition without obvious reason; the condition rapidly becomes continuous and severe and resistant to any form of treatment. Lacking knowledge as to the cause of these conditions, the treatment must be largely symptomatic. The prognosis is not good. These are usually called "intrinsic" allergies on the assumption that they are due to some condition which has developed within the body of the patient rather than from some allergen from the outside. Some allergists see a considerable number of patients who, they believe, belong in this group. Others find few of them. Climatic and other factors may make the difference.

A certain number of chronic recurrent headaches or allergic migraines are satisfactorily relieved by allergic management. Some of us believe that allergy accounts for a large percentage of these conditions and that treatment on this basis offers a satisfactory solution for these problems. There are, however, many causes of headache, and determination of an allergic basis for any particular case may be a matter of careful, painstaking investigation. Certainly it would seem that any headache which has resisted all other forms of treatment over a period of years deserves consideration as possibly due to allergy.

Not all cases of urticaria (hives, nettlerash) are of allergic origin. Focal infection and purely emotional factors account for a certain proportion. Furthermore these other factors may play a part in cases primarily associated with allergy. Even so, about 80 per cent of intermittent urticaria is relieved; 60 per cent of chronic urticaria.

The dermatologist (skin specialist) has a very pessimistic view of atopic eczema. He believes that the cause of the condition is seldom discovered and treatment is infrequently successful. The allergist is much more optimistic both as to finding an explanation for the eczema and also effecting definite relief. It must be admitted that in many instances the cause cannot be found, or may be found only after long and detailed investigation, and the result of treatment may not be all that is desired. This condition is one which requires, and deserves, patient investigation.

Contact dermatitis clears up rapidly if the contact excitant can be discovered and avoided. This may be simple or it may be very difficult. The substance responsible for the dermatitis may be something connected with the person's occupation and avoidance may mean the abandonment of a livelihood. If some method can be devised by which contact may be avoided, the person may continue his work and remain well. In the case of those sensitive to contact with flowers, weeds, or other forms of vegetation, hyposensitization is usually quite effective.

In nearly all forms of allergy, with the exception of intrinsic asthma which responds unsatisfactorily to all treatment the first 50 or 75 per cent of improvement is usually rapid and easily accomplished. The last 25 per cent is often slow and tedious. If the offending foods or environmental factors can be completely avoided then relief should be prompt and complete. If avoidance cannot be complete, treatment may bring about relief, but this requires considerable time and may not give absolute freedom from symptoms.

Cure

Allergists have some hesitancy in using the word "cure." They prefer to speak of relief. This is not because the patient cannot be apparently cured of the manifestation of the moment, but because the doctor realizes that the tendency is inherited and that symptoms may recur at some time in the future, due either to the development of new sensitizations or to the patient's becoming careless in his avoidance of the old offenders. It is not uncommon to hear a patient say that he had asthma or hay fever for a number of years then spontaneously lost it. After an interval of several years the same condition may recur and, in its recurrence, may or may not be due to the same allergen which caused the first allergic reactions. Apparent cures may prove to be real and permanent but many others are only periods of respite with a later recurrence. For this reason, it is impossible to know if and when a person is truly "cured."

For those in the lucky group listed above, those with adequate relief, no further message is needed. It is the unlucky minority, inclined to become discouraged before the sometimes long-drawn-out period of treatment has been completed, who will wish to know whether there is still a possibility that they may be transferred to the more fortunate category. For these our message continues. It would also be well for the lucky ones to continue to read, since the permanency of their good fortune depends upon continuous cooperation and an understanding of the problem with which they are faced.

Obstacles to Relief

Assuming that avoidance or desensitization or a combination of both has failed to provide relief within a reasonable period of time, let us analyze possible factors which have contributed to this failure.

1. *Failure to recognize an important allergen.* Skin tests are not infallible. An important test may have given a false negative reaction. Or, the doctor may not have tested with the proper allergen. In the past it has been considered necessary to test with a very large number of things in order that, by the very comprehensiveness of testing, one may be sure nothing of value is omitted. The tendency now is to do a much smaller number of tests but to select them with care. This requires the doctor to know the food habits of those living in the part of the country from which the patient comes and to make detailed inquiry into the eating habits of the patient. The doctor must know enough of the composition of foods to be able to determine if the patient gets certain foods without being aware of it. For example, the patient may deny the use of sage yet get it in considerable amount in sausage. He may get wheat flour in mayonnaise and Karaya gum in candy. It is not expected that the patient will have all this information but the doctor must if he is to do good work in allergy. Skin testing with foods may be sufficiently comprehensive without being too elaborate if proper judgment is used with adequate knowledge.

The physician attempts to learn from discussion as much as possible concerning the home environment of the patient, but unless he should have an opportunity to spend a day or longer in the home, there is much of which he must remain ignorant. A child's mother may assure the doctor that they have no pets at home, forgetting that the child spends some time each day frolicking with a dog belonging to his playmates. A young woman may tell her questioner all that is to be told of her home environment, her diet and the like, but finds herself tongue-tied when it comes to volunteering the information that her relationship with her husband is most strained and that she suspects him of infidelity, or that she herself has become infatuated with another woman's husband and that although she knows she is doing wrong she has been unable to find a satisfactory solution to her problem. Factors such as these are occasionally of importance in the solution of the problems of allergy.

Although the mistress of the home may consider herself the best of housekeepers, she cannot prevent dust from settling in the vents of a hot air heating system and being recirculated when the heat is turned on. Even a new house may have a damp cellar in which molds grow in abundance, unknown to the doctor and unrecognized by the patient.

The search for and removal of all offending allergens sometimes develop into a detective game. There is the story of two sea captains one of whom always had asthma while on the high seas, never while in port, while the second always suffered attacks within an hour or two after arrival at any port, being "immune" when at sea. The former was found sensitized to kapok, a relatively nonabsorbent fiber which is used in life preservers and often as the stuffing of pillows, especially on vessels. Whenever he lay down in his cabin he was exposed to kapok dust. The second was allergic to orris root, a constituent of many cosmetics. Evidently he lived true to the traditions of the sailor, on shore as afloat.

One reason for the writing of this book is to impress upon the victim of allergy the need for his having imagination and a disposition to inquire into possibilities, equally as much as the physician. The physician must depend upon him for many of the leads which facilitate ultimate success.

Many a doctor has had the experience, on greeting a new patient and asking "What's bothering you?" of receiving the terse reply, "That's for you to find out." The Chinese doctor solved this in an ingenious way. The tale is told that the Chinese patient never tells the doctor a thing. A Chinese physician, wise in the knowledge of the psychology of his race, explained how he acquired the necessary information. He was called to see a man, obviously suffering great pain. Asking no questions, he promptly announced that the patient had a pain in his back. The sick man grinned in triumph saying, "No, doctor, you are wrong, the pain is in my right knee." The physician then continued with the formula, replying, "Yes, of course the pain is in your right knee now, but it started in your back last night when you were asleep." The doctor had obtained the necessary information, following a route which was unnecessarily circuitous.

The allergic person who places all the responsibility on the doctor, who is not sufficiently interested in his own case to try to help solve the riddle, who does not recognize the need for cooperation to the last detail, and who is quite sure ultimately to place all blame for failure on his medical adviser, makes the solution of the problem doubly difficult, and often contributes to ultimate failure.

2. *Premature discouragement.* The victim of allergy should understand that his malady is essentially a chronic one. Since it is hereditary, he should realize that he was born with the allergic tendency, will carry it through life, and may transmit it to his offspring. The sensitization at a given period of his life may be adequately controlled, with consequent freedom from symptoms. At the same time he may be spontaneously developing some new sensitization which may cause return of symptoms in the future. He must resign himself to the realization that he may need professional advice, even treatment, for long periods and, at intervals, for possibly an indefinite period. The poorer the immediate results, the harder the doctor will have to work to achieve success and the more important is the need for intelligent cooperation by the patient.

Sensitization is usually multiple. If there are, let us say, 12 allergenic factors active in a given case and 10 are discovered, best results will not accrue until the additional 2 have been identified. Time is often necessary for its accomplishment.

In the writer's experience there are two periods during which chronic allergics tend to become discouraged and wish to discontinue treatment. These are during the second and third months and at the end of one year. Since the vast majority show quite satisfactory improvement almost from the beginning, those who do not have this fortunate experience and who had expected the doctor to accomplish wonders almost at once become impatient and, discarding all of the advantages gained by the allergic diagnostic study and the first assay at treatment, "throw in the sponge" and dash off in search of some will-o'-the-wisp of promised speedy cure such as those found in the advertising pages of many magazines and newspapers.

One should realize that even though results may not be satisfactory at the end of a month or two, it does not mean that we are doomed to failure. A woman had her diagnostic study in early June. Her complaint was of perennial asthma with attacks coming so frequently that it was impossible to establish any seasonal variation. She was directed to avoid the use of feather pillows and exposure to feathers and house dust in so far as possible, and was given an appropriate dietary routine. Since she had given a positive reaction to ragweed she was advised that in the event of exacerbation of symptoms during the ragweed season in August and September, she should report the fact so that coseasonal treatment could be administered. She was next seen in mid-October, when she was completely discouraged, announcing that the treatment had failed entirely. She readily admitted that at the beginning she had been most hopeful, since from early June to mid-August she had been fully 80 per cent relieved. From then on and until about a week prior to the second consultation, her symptoms had been as bad as ever. It was pointed out that the return of symptoms was in all probability due to ragweed pollen, and that she should have reported the recurrence. Under any circumstance the pollen season was now over and she could look forward with assurance to rapid improvement and continued relief until the next ragweed season, with no change whatsoever in the program of treatment. The following year and on succeeding years she was hyposensitized prior to the ragweed season and for a number of years has now maintained her 80 per cent relief.

It is experiences such as these which have led the allergist to advise his patients that they must keep in close touch with him for at least a year, through the twelve months, since different factors may play a part at different seasons of the year. The first year of treatment in the chronic persistent case is a period of orientation in which the patient's reaction to seasonal and other factors is being observed. This will serve as the basis for the more permanent therapeutic program.

It is a good plan, if there is not marked improvement within the first three months, to go over the situation with the physician to see if any explanation can be found for the failure to improve. Whether one is depending on avoidance or hyposensitization or both for relief, three months is long enough to wait for definite improvement.

The patient recalls something having been said about a year of treatment, through the four seasons, and, in the face of failure after the first twelve months, he is likely to become discouraged. There might be some argument as to whether one could call this premature discouragement. Certainly within a year one should commence to see at least a modicum of results. Most persons do, in fact have done so long before the expiration of the year. Others who have not, but who have intelligently followed the analysis of the causative factors in the different months of the first year, can see the logic of anticipating better results in the second year.

At the same time failure of any improvement within a year makes it less probable that success will ultimately be achieved and one can therefore readily understand discouragement at the end of this interval.

There are many who, looking back upon ten or twenty years of illness, unhesitatingly announce that a year or two or even several years of treatment will be well worth the effort if in the end they are saved from perpetuation of the experiences of the preceding decades.

One should not become discouraged at the end of one or even two or three months. One should not become discouraged at the end of a year. When, then, if at any time, may the poor patient have the privilege of becoming discouraged, without being accused of prematurity? The reader who has followed the logic of the preceding paragraphs will readily realize that there must follow a logical time for becoming discouraged. This is at the end of the second year. That is the time to consider a change of doctors or a change in therapeutic methods.

Those who have on the other hand achieved a clearly recognized measure of relief, even though it be but partial, should not stop treatment at the end of the second year. They should plan on continuing for as many years as may be necessary, with reasonable assurance of continued gradual improvement in the course of time. Fortunately, as time passes, treatment usually becomes less strenuous and more simplified. Desensitizing injections given at the beginning at intervals of from three to seven days are eventually spaced at intervals of from two to four weeks, many of the dietary proscriptions are abrogated, and one often finds that eventually he may eat offending foods or experience exposure to other allergens in moderate concentration, on occasion, even though he might not tolerate them as a daily routine (see Chart I on page 111).

3. *Unavoidable contingencies.* The two preceding groups of factors interfering with success are not insurmountable, provided the patient and doctor both have enough intellectual curiosity to attempt to work out the problem in collaboration and provided sufficient time is allowed for this purpose. We now come to the truly unfortunate class of allergics, those who are unimproved after two years. Any one or a combination of several obstacles may interfere with relief.

Even though the number of allergenic excitants for a given case may not be great, under certain circumstances it may be impossible to avoid all of them completely. This is noted in such conditions as occupational dermatitis and in food allergy when one must eat in restaurants where adequate culinary control is impracticable.

Other pathologic states within the body of the allergic may interfere with recovery. This applies more particularly to focal infection with or without bacterial sensitization, and possibly also to endocrine disturbances, derangement of the glands of internal secretion. Whether or not one be sensitized to germs living and growing in a focus of infection such as the sinuses, dental root abscesses, tonsils, gall bladder, etc., this type of infection may interfere with good results.

Secondary changes may have occurred as a result of long-standing allergic responses, changes which are not reversible. A characteristic of the allergic response is that the reaction is reversible, that the tissues may return completely to normal after the excitant has ceased to act. However, long-standing asthma may result in certain chest deformities which are permanent and which result in lasting shortness of breath, which the patient may interpret as asthma. It may result in chronic infection of the bronchial tree, a bronchitis, or bronchiectasis which, once it has developed, must be cured, if possible, entirely independently of the allergic treatment. Long-standing edema or water-logging of the mucous membranes of the nose predisposes to infection of the sinuses. The latter may persist long after the hay fever or nasal allergy has been relieved. There is evidence that certain changes may occur in blood vessels as a result of long-standing allergic response, which are irreversible and represent permanent damage.

Although other factors may play a part in the prevention of relief, those discussed in these three categories account for the vast majority of failures. In addition, it needs to be said that there is an occasional case in which no adequate explanation can be found in spite of the most careful search by the trained allergist and the most satisfactory cooperation of the patient. This is particularly true of the "intrinsic" asthmatic in whom we usually fail to find the cause of the asthma. But there is also the occasional patient in whom the diagnostic findings seem adequately to explain the condition and in whom treatment is carried out in the approved manner, yet who does not get satisfactory relief. Why, we do not know.

No War Is Won

Military strategists have said that no war is won. The victor finds himself little better off than the vanquished. In a slightly different sense we may say that the war of allergy is never won, since with the inherited allergic predisposition, and the consequent tendency to become sensitized to environmental and similar factors, even though one has apparently been cured, the possibility always remains that new sensitizations may develop. Fortunately, however, there is definite evidence that if one is protected from contact with offending allergens the tendency to develop new sensitizations is diminished, except among those few in whom the inheritance is of an extreme degree. This justifies the statement that treatment should be commenced early, before symptoms have persisted long and sensitization has become multiple, and that the more effectively the treatment is applied, the less probability will there be that symptoms will recur at some time in the future. The cumulative experience of many victims of the malady indicates clearly that what may for all purposes be designated "cure" is possible. Avoidance for a sufficiently long period may result in loss of sensitization and treatment over a long period often will bring about permanent relief. We have seen a number of patients suffering from seasonal hay fever who, after several seasons of treatment, could remain well without further treatment. The number of these is sufficiently greater than of those who could expect spontaneous cure to make the figure statistically significant. With a decreasing number of sensitizations and decreasing frequency of attacks, the probability of new sensitizations and recurrent attacks progressively diminishes.

There remains the hope, not yet achieved, that some day some scientist may solve the whole secret of allergic sensitization, producing a drug or other remedy which will effectively organize the State of Allergy so that it no longer goes into violent commotion following the sudden appearance of an enemy within its borders. Until then we must continue with the present method, the detection of every individual marauder and the selection of appropriate methods for protection against each of them as they come to the fore.

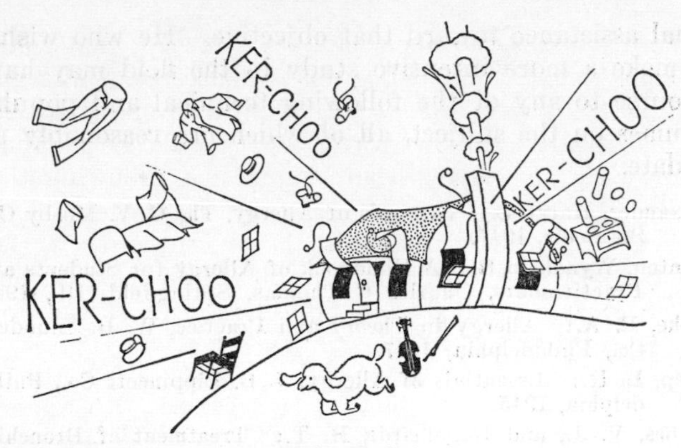

Hold Tight!

XII

GENERAL ORDERS—DIRECTIONS TO THE PATIENT

Not many years ago doctors who wished to learn of the new developments in the field of allergy were under the impression that they could do so by taking a week off from their regular work in which to visit some allergy clinic. Today it is quite generally recognized that an adequate postgraduate training in the subject requires at least a year of intensive study.

The same applies to those persons who are subject to attacks which are allergic in nature. There is no universal short cut to cure through self-medication. This little volume has not been written in the hope that the reader will, upon its completion, be so well informed on the subject that he can cure himself. The nature of the malady renders it quite impracticable. It has been written solely so that the victim of the disease may acquire sufficient understanding of his problem so that he can understand what the doctor is endeavoring to accomplish and can give the physician his own personal assistance toward that objective. He who wishes to make a more intensive study in the field may have recourse to any of the following technical and popular volumes on the subject, all of which are reasonably up to date.

Alexander, Harry L.: Synopsis of Allergy, The C. V. Mosby Co., St. Louis, 1947.

Blanton, Wyndham B.: A Handbook of Allergy for Students and Practitioners, Charles C Thomas, Springfield, Ill., 1942.

Cooke, R. A.: Allergy in Theory and Practice, W. B. Saunders Co., Philadelphia, 1947.

Criep, L. H.: Essentials of Allergy, J. B. Lippincott Co., Philadelphia, 1945.

Derbes, V. J., and Engelhardt, H. T.: Treatment of Bronchial Asthma, J. B. Lippincott Co., Philadelphia, 1946.

Durham, O. C.: Your Hay Fever, Bobbs-Merrill Co., Indianapolis, 1936.

Feinberg, Samuel M.: Allergy in Practice, Year Book Publishers, Chicago, 1946.

Hansel, French K.: Clinical Allergy, The C. V. Mosby Co., St. Louis, 1953.

Ratner, Bret: Allergy, Anaphylaxis and Immunotherapy, Williams and Wilkins Co., Baltimore, 1943.

Rowe, Albert H.: Elimination Diets and the Patient's Allergies, Lea & Febiger, Philadelphia, 1944.

Sheldon, J. M., Lovell, R. G., and Mathews, K. P.: A Manual of Clinical Allergy, W. B. Saunders Co., Philadelphia, 1953.

Sulzberger, Marion B.: Dermatologic Allergy, Charles C Thomas, Springfield, Ill., 1940.

Tuft, Louis: Clinical Allergy, Lea & Febiger, Philadelphia, 1949.

Unger, Leon: Bronchial Asthma, Charles C Thomas, Springfield, Ill., 1945.

Urbach, Erich, and Gottlieb, Philip: Allergy, Grune and Stratton, New York, 1946.

Vaughan and Black: Practice of Allergy, The C. V. Mosby Co., St. Louis, 1954.

Vaughan, Warren T.: Strange Malady. The Story of Allergy, Doubleday, Doran & Co., Inc., New York, 1941.

Miscellaneous Instructions

The following miscellaneous instructions have been formulated to aid persons with one or another of the manifestations of allergy. The reader who has allergy will find no difficulty in determining those instructions which apply to his individual case, although of course the physician will designate those which are to be followed.

General Instructions

Allergy is in great measure very much of a chronic malady. In the great majority of cases it is hereditary in that the tendency to become sensitized to one or another allergen is inherited. Since we cannot alter the allergic inheritance our effort must be to find the exciting causes (nonhereditary) and remove them insofar as possible. When this is successful symptoms are completely relieved, but the hereditary tendency persists. It occasionally happens, therefore, that a person even when under treatment becomes sensitized to some new substance. This complicates the picture and requires that we keep in fairly close touch with you for a period sufficiently long to be sure that you are going to be relieved and stay relieved. Furthermore, it is very desirable that we follow your case carefully through the four seasons, for at least a year, since different allergenic substances are active at different times of the year. This applies especially to pollens and to foods, but also applies to certain other allergenic substances. We would therefore like you to report by letter concerning your condition at intervals of from four to six weeks throughout the first year following the examination. From the information which you furnish we will be able to advise you and your physician concerning any changes in the treatment or concerning further treatment. It is very important that you furnish these reports regularly, no matter whether you are doing splendidly or not doing well. If we have given you any extract or medicine for desensitization, please notify us when you have used it up so that we may advise you concerning further treatment. Please remember that if you are going to obtain the best results and most permanent results, you must keep us informed as to how you are doing; you must cooperate wholeheartedly in following the treatment exactly as it is prescribed, and in avoiding things that should be avoided, absolutely, completely; and you must notify us without delay if there is a return of symptoms, no matter when this occurs.

General Directions for a Patient with Pollen Hay Fever or Pollen Asthma

1. You have been tested with the various pollens and have been found sensitized to certain of these. Some are pollens which are not carried great distances through the air and can therefore be fairly easily avoided. Others are wind-borne and cannot be

avoided. For relief you must therefore be desensitized with those which have been shown actually to cause the symptoms in your case. Not every pollen which gives positive skin reactions necessarily causes symptoms.

2. The best time to start desensitization treatment is now. In other words it makes no difference at what time during the year treatment is inaugurated, but the earlier it is begun the better will be your results. For example, if "now" happens to be in the middle of a pollen season you will ask the question, Is it worth while to take the treatment this early? The answer is Yes, you should start now. Treatment will probably give you a good measure of relief for this season and now is the time to start for next season, continuing with perennial desensitization throughout the year. Indeed, "now" is the time to start even for year after next! The total number of injections is no greater with perennial treatment than with preseasonal desensitization. The intervals between injections are increased.

3. Be sure to report regularly for your treatment, as often as directed by your physician. If you wait too long between treatments the degree of your hyposensitization will drop somewhat and the doctor will have to decrease the strength of his next injection, thereby losing some of the advantage gained. The interval between injections varies, depending on how much time we have before the next pollen season and upon the degree to which your tolerance has been increased.

4. When you go to your doctor for treatment, always carry with you two or three, three-eighths grain or three-fourth grain ephedrine capsules, to be taken by mouth in the event you develop a reaction following treatment (hives, sneezing, or asthma). In the event you develop such a reaction, take a capsule at once and report without delay to your physician, who will give you the proper medicine for prompt relief. If after taking the ephedrine your symptoms are not improving within ten minutes, take another capsule and apply a tight band around the arm above the place where you received your injection.

5. You should stay in the doctor's office thirty minutes after each treatment since, if reaction occurs, it will usually occur within this time. Hives sometimes appear a couple of hours later but are relieved by taking one or two ephedrine capsules.

6. One is more likely to develop a reaction if one undertakes strenuous exercise or gets overheated within the first two or three hours after injection. Therefore avoid both of these.

7. The relief that you will experience during the pollen season will depend in great measure upon the thoroughness with which you have been desensitized. You may have no symptoms what-

soever, but usually in each pollen season there are two or three or more peak days in which the pollen concentration of the air is unusually heavy, so heavy that you may have symptoms. But this rarely totals more than five or six days in any season.

8. In the event your relief is only partial it is possible to procure a pollen filter which may be placed in the window of your bedroom. This ventilates the room with air from which most of the pollen has been removed. Where desensitization is not complete it may be possible to spend your eight sleeping hours in such an atmosphere and tolerate the daylight hours better because of the comfortable night.

9. When desensitization is only partially successful it may be that this failure of complete relief is due to your being allergic, at the same time, to some of the foods that you are eating or to some other allergens. Therefore, if you are not entirely relieved, inquire of your doctor whether you should go on any specific dietary restrictions or avoid other substances such as orris root, face powder, feathers, etc., during the pollen season. Such an avoidance will probably lessen the metabolic overload sufficiently so that you will be relieved of your pollen symptoms (see illustration on page 93).

10. If your eyes are very irritated your doctor can give you a prescription for eye drops which will relieve them. The following prescription is very helpful and can be formulated by your physician.

Adrenalin 1/1000—4 c.c.
Boric acid (saturated solution)—12 c.c.

Neo-Synephrine ¼ per cent or a solution of Antistine may be used as eye drops; these usually give a great deal of comfort.

11. If your nose is too stuffy or too "runny," your doctor may prescribe drops or a spray or give you a prescription for capsules or tablets which will help to keep the nose open and reduce the secretion. Ephedrine, Propadrine, Neo-Synephrine, Privine, and some of the "antihistamine" drugs may be used as a nasal spray or drops and Benzedrine may be used as an inhalant. Some of us prefer drugs by mouth since they act to shrink the swollen mucous membrane without causing any local irritation and because they cause a more complete action upon the entire surface of the mucous membrane. For this purpose we may use ephedrine, Neo-Synephrine, Propadrine, or one of the many "antihistamine" drugs. Some persons find one drug superior while others get more relief from another. When using a solution in the nose, after putting drops in each nostril, bend your head down forward between the knees so that the drops will run "upward" into the upper front part of the nose.

12. Avoid all unnecessary exposures to pollen. Do not take unnecessary or long rides through the country during the pollen season.

13. Have no cut flowers of any description in your house.

14. See that weeds or grasses in the vicinity of your house are cut before they have a chance to pollinate. They should be cut repeatedly. If you are allergic to grasses, do not mow your own lawn.

15. Cold, raw air irritates the mucous membranes. This is one reason why so many people sleeping with windows open awaken around three or four o'clock in the morning with symptoms. Therefore, do not sleep in drafts or on open sleeping porches. If the window must be open do not have cross ventilation if it can be avoided. A wet sheet hung a foot inside the open window will stop some of the pollen. If the windows are kept closed the air may be kept in circulation by an electric fan and this will add to your comfort but it should not be directed over your bed. The windows should be closed in the day time as well as at night.

16. If your doctor has been able to give you only partial relief, dark glasses will often help the hay fever symptoms.

17. Avoid constipation.

18. Do not over-eat. Your evening meal especially should be a light one.

19. Do not bathe in small swimming pools. You might develop sinusitis.

20. Do not dive in any water. This might produce sinus trouble.

21. Don't take cold baths. Take them warm or hot.

General Instructions for a Patient with Asthma or Vasomotor Rhinitis

In the preceding section we have discussed the general treatment of nasal and bronchial allergy when due to pollens. This section applies to nasal and bronchial allergy due to other causes. The symptoms are more likely to be present off and on throughout the year. However, patients with respiratory allergy due to either group of causes will do well to study carefully both sections.

1. You have been found allergic to certain allergens which appear to be responsible in part at least for your trouble. There may be other allergenic causes which have not yet been discovered. One of your duties will therefore be to make a careful study of your attacks and suggest to your doctor any other special factors which may occur to you.

2. Avoid those things which your doctor has told you to avoid, as thoroughly and completely as possible.

3. If your doctor has placed you on dietary avoidance, make the avoidance complete. Do not discontinue your diet if you are not promptly relieved, for some time must often elapse before you will experience recognizable results. Furthermore, it may be that there are other allergenic factors not yet discovered. In order to discover them you must carefully avoid those things which have already been found. If you return to contact with one of the known allergens it will make it more difficult finally to discover the unknown one.

4. Remember that contact with small amounts of an allergen is almost as bad as contact with large amounts. You should therefore make your avoidances absolute.

5. Certain substances are so frequently allergenic that you would do well to avoid them even though you are not now sensitized to them. It is the best way to prevent becoming sensitized to them at some time in the future. The following instructions apply in this regard.

6. You should have no animal pets.

7. You should have no flowers or plants in the house.

8. Keep your home as free from dust as possible. Once your house is made as dust-free as possible, keep it that way. If possible you should not do the dusting yourself.

9. Your bedroom particularly should be free from dust and from dust-catching articles. The floors should be cleaned and should be smooth so that they can be kept clean. There should be no heavy rugs or draperies and no upholstered furniture. Small wash rugs and wash curtains are allowable. Preparations are available, under the names Dust Seal and Allergex, for use on fabrics such as rugs, chair and divan covers, to prevent the escape of dust from them. From experience with these agents, it appears that they do no harm to fabrics and aid considerably in the control of house dust.

10. Your mattress and pillows should have dustproof covers. These are on the market.

11. Avoid insect powders and sprays in your home. If you must use insecticides use those that do not contain pyrethrum.

12. Avoid contact with feathers or the inhalation of feather dust.

13. The environment least likely to be allergenic for you is that of a relatively new house or apartment, well ventilated and with a proper heating system, hot water or steam, not hot air, and without upholstered furniture or heavy rugs or draperies. A hospital room serves as a good example.

14. In so far as possible avoid irritating smokes, odors, and perfumes. Leaky gas stoves, leaky electric refrigerators, oil lamps, odors from garages, fresh paint and varnish and the like are best avoided.

15. Avoid constipation. Do not use laxatives containing phenolphthalein. Your physician will instruct you regarding these. Children's asthmatic attacks are sometimes relieved by enemas.

16. Do not overload the stomach. All meals should be relatively light, especially the evening meal. Foods and beverages that produce gas, such as carbonated water, ginger ale and the like, should be avoided. If you are having asthma you will do well to stay on a liquid diet for a day or two and to drink warm or hot drinks, not cold drinks.

17. Avoid fatigue, strenuous exercise, emotional conflicts, and worry.

18. As you improve, do not let up on the stringency of your regulations until told to do so by your physician.

For information regarding medication, see Chapter X.

General Directions to a Patient with Allergic Eczema

1. What has been stressed concerning specific dietary restrictions in the two preceding sections applies equally here.

2. Avoid constipation. See that the bowels move daily. Do not use laxatives containing phenolphthalein. Your physician will tell you of these.

3. Do not overeat.

4. Avoid mechanical irritation of the affected skin. Scratch as little as possible.

5. Until told to do so by your doctor, do not allow water to touch the eczematous areas. Pure olive oil may be used for cleansing purposes.

6. Eat regularly and chew your food thoroughly.

7. Drink plenty of water. The amount to be used in your particular case should be prescribed by your physician.

8. Your doctor will prescribe any tonic that may be necessary.

9. Soothing lotions or ointments for external application may be prescribed. Since these may cause contact dermatitis in certain cases, you should first be patch-tested with them.

10. Sometimes dermatitis is due to dietary excess in fats or proteins or carbohydrates. If you do not respond on specific dietary restrictions, your doctor will modify the diet to control these various factors.

11. Your doctor will decide concerning the desirability of ultraviolet light treatment or x-ray treatment.

12. Don't forget that food allergy is not the only allergy which may be responsible for an allergic dermatitis. Feathers, wool, house dust, and many other contact or inhalant substances may be responsible. Study your contact exposures yourself and see if you can make some helpful suggestions to your doctor.

13. Don't forget that nonspecific factors may be playing a part. The clearing up of focal infection and the improvement of your general health is most important.

14. Above all remember that fatigue will usually make an eczema worse. See that you get plenty of rest, both physical and mental.

15. All soaps are naturally irritating and are better not used in eczematous areas. Certainly no brands of soap should be used without preliminary patch testing with a dilute solution thereof.

The ''antihistamine'' drugs frequently give much relief from itching both when taken internally and when used in ointments for local application. They seem to have no effect on the healing of the eczema but they may contribute a great deal to your comfort. Some of these are very good sensitizers themselves so they should be used with care and continued observation to make sure that the remedy itself may not contribute to the continuance of the eczema.

Hydrocortisone acetate ointment in one or two and one-half per cent concentration often gives very prompt relief from itching and great improvement in the eczema. For contact eczemas which clear up promptly when the cause is discovered and avoided, hydrocortisone is very helpful in cutting short the discomfort and disability. In chronic eczemas the effect is only temporary and the condition recurs as soon as the drug is stopped, but it is very helpful during a period of acute exacerbation.

General Directions for a Person with Allergic Headache

1. Much that has been said in the preceding sections will apply in the directions to a victim of allergic headache.

2. Remember that allergy is but one factor in the intricate mechanism responsible for your disease. Your doctor will take other factors into consideration in the event you do not progress satisfactorily on simple allergic avoidances.

3. Avoid fatigue, both physical and mental. This is even more important than in the case of allergic eczema.

4. Avoid emotional excitement.

5. If your attacks are associated in any way with your periods, tell your doctor.

6. If there is any regular periodicity to your attacks, which often is the case, tell your doctor and study your case yourself to see if you can discover any possible cause that has a chance to act only periodically.

7. Keep a food diary.

8. If you do not progress satisfactorily, your doctor may put you on an elimination diet.

9. He will give you the proper medicines for avoiding attacks if possible and for relief of pain during the attack.

10. Sometimes the nervous element is very important. Even though you may consider yourself not at all a nervous individual and may feel that you have no mental problems to cope with, it is sometimes advisable to call in a competent psychiatrist to collaborate in the treatment of your type of condition.

Urticaria and Angioneurotic Edema

In general these same instructions apply to patients suffering from recurrent or chronic urticaria or angioneurotic edema. The "antihistamine" drugs are usually quite successful in controlling the wheals and swellings in these conditions and in relief of the itching.

Instructions to a Patient With Allergic Colitis or Indigestion

1. While you have been found allergic to certain foods and must avoid them completely as instructed by your physician, you should bear in mind that there are other factors than allergy which are responsible for your condition. The more important of these are covered in the following.

2. You should avoid constipation. At the same time very active cathartics should be avoided. If possible you should secure daily evacuations without laxatives, by taking a bland, nonirritating diet.

3. If you require laxatives it is better to use plain salt enemas, two teaspoonfuls of ordinary salt to a quart of lukewarm water. Do not use any laxatives containing phenolphthalein or other laxatives that stimulate the large bowel. Obtain instructions from your physician.

4. Bulky or roughage foods should be avoided. While these may temporarily lessen the tendency to constipation they will eventually cause increased trouble. For this reason avoid vege-

tables containing much fiber, bran, whole wheat bread, Graham bread, brown bread and the like.

5. Vegetables containing fiber may be passed through a sieve or colander to remove the fiber. Such puréed canned vegetables may be purchased from your grocer. These are usually sold as baby foods. Among the ready prepared fruits and vegetables which are available at your grocer's in this form are puréed spinach, carrots, asparagus, tomatoes, prunes, beans, peas, beets, apicrot pulp, squash.

6. On a rigid, nonresidue diet you may be allowed the following foods.

Cream of wheat or rice	Coffee
Lean meat	Cocoa
Roast breast of chicken	Chocolate
Fish	Angel food
Irish potato	Sponge cake
Puréed vegetables	Ice cream
Tomato juice	Sherbets
Strained broth	Orange (juice only)
Strained cream soups	Custards
Asparagus (tips only)	Blanc mange
Lettuce	Jellies
White bread	Farina
Crackers	Corn flakes
Eggs	Rice
Milk	Macaroni
Cream cheese	Spaghetti
Tea	Noodles

7. Any of these foods to which you have been found allergic must, of course, be avoided. Your doctor will advise you concerning any other food that you may take.

8. Lie down for one-half hour after each meal with local heat to the abdomen (hot water bottle or electric pad).

9. It should be ascertained whether you have any organic disturbance of the gastrointestinal tract which requires treatment along with the treatment of your abdominal allergy. This may or may not require x-ray studies. If you have some visceroptosis (sagging of the abdominal organs) this may also require adjustment and treatment.

10. If your symptoms come in attacks, you should keep a food diary.

11. Your doctor will give you the necessary medicines.

12. If you do not notice immediate improvement, do not be discouraged, because so many different factors interact that it sometimes takes time to discover and remove all of the causes.

Sometimes weeks or even months of supervision are necessary before complete relief is obtained.

Directions for Avoiding and Removing House Dust

1. Renovate the house or room, but while this is being done, *you* keep away. We have seen dust allergics thoughtlessly go home to get the dust out of the house themselves!

2. Take down all draperies, curtains, hangings. Take up all rugs.

3. Either send them to be cleaned or have them cleaned outside the house. A vacuum cleaner, dry cleaning, and soap and water do wonderfully.

4. Remove all pictures and other dust catchers. Wash what may be washed and clean the remainder with a damp or oiled cloth. Store away until cleaning is finished.

5. Clean the picture molding with oiled cloth, and dust down the walls. Hot air heating is not satisfactory. Seal such flues, also other holes where dust might enter.

6. Go over all furniture with oiled cloth or damp cloth—top, bottom, front, back, inside, and outside. Pay especial attention to bed springs and slats, rear of chiffoniers and chifforobes, etc. Cover furniture with sheets until remainder of cleaning is completed.

In your bedroom use plain iron and wooden furniture that can be washed each week. Do not use box springs unless covered with a dustproof cover. All bedclothes must be washed each week. It may later be necessary to cover the mattress with a specially made envelope of rubber sheeting or fabricoid. Most large department stores now carry dustproof pillow and mattress covers.

7. Wash down woodwork, floors, radiators, etc.

8. After things are again set up, it is best to have no heavy rugs, in the bedrooms at least, and only such draperies as may be washed. Rag rugs and draperies are to be washed once weekly.

9. Try to keep it that way!

10. Vacuum cleaning may be allowed, but not dry sweeping. If a broom must be used, sprinkle torn bits of paper soaked in water generously over the floor before starting.

11. Allow no animals in the house.

12. Look to see if there are damp, moldy, mildewy areas in the house (kitchen, bathroom, cellar, ceiling), and if so report to the doctor. He may then want to test you with molds.

13. Regardless of how thoroughly one may clean the house or how consistently cleaning is continued, it is impossible to keep the house sufficiently free of dust to make hyposensitiza-

tion unnecessary. Although meticulous care may be used to maintain scrupulous cleanliness, treatment with dust extract is always necessary. Since this is true, it has always seemed to us unwise to require onerous and time-consuming effort on the part of the housekeeper. If she, by her efforts, could obviate the necessity of hyposensitization, it would be justifiable but, since she cannot, we think it best to be satisfied with good housekeeping and then depend largely upon treatment. In our hands, this has given satisfactory results. In those needing additional help, Allergex and Dust Seal are helpful.

Dust Seal or Allergex may be used to treat rugs, carpets, and upholstered furniture. This will make it unnecessary to do away with these furnishings and make the care of them much easier.

Since hyposensitization to dust is always necessary in true dust sensitivity regardless of the effort made to maintain a dust-free home, it does not seem reasonable to demand onerous, time-consuming, constantly recurring efforts to keep the house dust free. Good housekeeping with proper treatment for the sensitivity is all that need be required except in the extreme case.

Directions for the Avoidance of Feathers

There are very few homes in which feathers are not widely distributed through most of the rooms. Feather pillows are in the bedroom, also often "down" comforts, and occasionally, feather beds. Overstuffed furniture in the bedroom or living room sometimes contains some feathers. Canary birds and occasionally parrots may be a source of feather dust.

In extremely reactive cases it sometimes becomes necessary to remove all feathers completely from the house. As a rule, however, it is only necessary to render the bedroom completely free from feathers and feather dust. This provides about eight hours during which the patient is free from contact with feather dust and this is usually enough, especially if the patient is at the same time receiving desensitization with feather extract, to enable him to tolerate the small amount of exposure that he will experience elsewhere during the day.

All feathers must be removed from the bedroom. Pillows should not be stored in an adjoining closet since the dust from gradually disintegrating feathers slowly permeates the closet and seeps out into the room when the door is opened.

A cotton, kapok or silk floss, or rubber foam pillow may be substituted for the feather pillow. Unfortunately an allergic individual tends to become sensitized to kapok after prolonged exposure. Therefore it may be better to cover the feather pillow with a dustproof slip.

Inexpensive dustproof pillow covers may be obtained from all large department stores. Your doctor will be able to tell you where to procure them. An ordinary pillow slip may be put on over the dustproof cover.

Feather dust becomes generally distributed throughout any bedroom. This consists of small, microscopic particles of the scale from feathers which can be easily seen if one will shake a feather pillow in a shaft of sunlight as it comes in through the window. It therefore becomes important to make the bedroom as free from dust as possible and thereafter to keep it that way. All dust catchers and dust makers should be removed from the bedroom.

Directions for Those Sensitive to Cosmetics

Until recently orris root has been used in cosmetics and perfumes because, acting as a mordant, it helped to retain the pleasant odor.

Now orris has been dispensed with and powders and creams generally are free of it. Some orris oil is used in other preparations, but there is considerable question as to whether this will cause any trouble. This means that the greatest source of trouble in cosmetics has been removed and cosmetics are not the important source of trouble they once were. You may be sensitive to something else in powder, so cosmetics cannot be entirely forgotten in the search for the cause of your trouble, and it is still helpful to have powders and other cosmetics which are as free as can be made of all things which usually cause trouble. Among those generally available and quite satisfactory are Almay, Ar-Ex, Ethix, Frost, Luzier, Mansfield, and Marcelle.

Lipstick, creams, even rouge and powder, may cause a dermatitis due to some constituent to which you may be sensitive. By carefully investigating the matter you should be able to find a preparation which you can use without any irritation.

Directions for the Avoidance of Pyrethrum

Pyrethrum, which is derived from the petals of a species of chrysanthemum, is widely used as an insecticide in insect powders and sprays. It is related to the active agent in ragweed pollen, so those sensitive to ragweed usually are disturbed by pyrethrum and it should be carefully avoided. DDT has come into quite general use and is a very effective agent which causes little trouble. "Cedarene" is quite satisfactory. Paradichlorobenzene cakes, in perforated tins, may be hung in closets to repel moths. They contain no pyrethrum.

Discussion of Avoidance of Wheat, Egg, and Milk

The three food substances which are most widely used in our modern dietary and which are called for in the largest number of recipes are wheat, egg, and milk. Bread was a wonderful discovery back in prehistoric times, because it indicated that man had discovered a way of storing food (in the form of flour) for use during those periods of the year when fresh food was not available. In this sense it was indeed the staff of life. Today, with all of the facilities that are available for procuring fresh foods at any time of year or for preserving and storing almost any type of food, wheat flour and bread are no longer essential parts of the diet. One could live as well and as long without any wheat at all.

Milk is more nearly the perfect food than any other single food, and is almost essential for proper development of the growing infant. Substitute food combinations have, however, been perfected in which all the necessary elements for normal growth are provided. Nutramigen and the soy bean substitutes, Mull-Soy and So-Bee, contain all the required nutritive substances, and children can be kept on these substitutes for months with no deleterious effect. Growth and nutrition proceed normally. Strained meat formulas have been devised and are quite satisfactory. One is on the market prepared by a purveyor of "baby foods."

Heating milk does not always change it enough to make it nonallergic. Ratner states that milk needs to be boiled three to six hours to be made nonallergic and that evaporated milk should be boiled several minutes.

Some persons who cannot take cow's milk will tolerate goat's milk. In most cities of moderate or large size there are good goat dairies where fresh goat's milk may be procured. These are supervised by the health authorities and meet the same requirements for cleanliness as cow dairies. When fresh goat's milk may not be found, good canned milk is usually available and serves the purpose perfectly well.

The avoidance of wheat, egg, or milk and more particularly the avoidance of two or even three, entails considerable inconvenience because they are so widely used in the preparation of such a large number of dishes. One eating away from home is often in a quandary concerning probable constituents of this or that culinary preparation. Since so much that is in the modern cookbook is inappropriate, many special recipes have been devised to provide substitute dishes for those who must avoid one or more of these basic foods.

It seems unnecessary to incorporate such recipes in this volume, not so much because of the large amount of space that they would take, but rather because they are so readily available elsewhere. Pamphlets containing large numbers of substitute food recipes may be obtained at small cost from The Bureau of Home Economics, United States Department of Agriculture, Washington. Rowe's *Elimination Diets and Patients' Allergies,* Tuft's *Clinical Allergy,* and Vaughan's *Practice of Allergy* all contain large numbers of substitute recipes. These sources may be consulted by those whose sensitizations are such as to require substitutions. Stores supplying nonallergic foods can supply recipes for various purposes and the makers of "substitute" foods can supply recipes on request.

The writer's experience has been, however, that most persons in this group prefer not to take the trouble to prepare special dishes. In the majority of homes today, even the bread is prepared outside, in the bakery, and no one is especially interested in making a special bread for just one member of the family. The majority therefore avoid what they must, and otherwise eat the same dishes as their neighbors, possibly with some broadening by the inclusion of varieties of foods which were not previously being eaten. Suggestions for additional foods that may be used in this way appear in the tables which follow.

Some of those allergic to wheat are allergic also to rye but there are those who can eat rye bread without ill result. The rye bread usually found at the bakery or the grocery contains a considerable amount of wheat flour and is not a satisfactory replacement for wheat bread. Pure rye bread is difficult to make into a satisfactory loaf and most bakers do not want to be bothered with making it, particularly when the sale is not large. In moderate-sized and larger cities there is usually some one place where a pure rye bread may be found. Ry-Krisp crackers and Horlamus Rye Bread* have national distribution and are entirely satisfactory.

Various flours are available, such as lima bean, soy bean, potato, rice, rye, barley, and others, and recipes for using them in the preparation of cakes, cookies, griddle cakes, and bread are available. Safemix is a mixture of soy and potato flour.

Corn bread, rye bread and buckwheat cakes as usually prepared contain some wheat flour and cannot be used.

---

*Ry-Krisp, The Ralston Purina Company, St. Louis. This is available in most restaurants. Horlamus Rye Bread, (Hypo Allergic Foods, N. Irene Horlamus, Director, 215 S. W. 42nd Avenue, P. O. Box 1712, Riverside Station, Miami, Florida) is shipped in vacuum sealed tins and retains its freshness for at least eight months. Ry-Krisp contains no wheat, egg, or milk. Horlamus bread contains only pure rye flour, cottonseed shortening and yeast.

Directions for Wheat Avoidance

In eliminating wheat it is necessary to avoid it completely, since small amounts are as likely to produce symptoms as are large amounts. The following pure flours may be purchased through your grocer or from the Chicago Dietetic Supply House, 1750 West Van Buren Street, Chicago, Ill. On request they will send you a price list and recipes:

- Potato starch
- Rye flour
- Pure buckwheat
- Cornstarch
- Barley flour
- Rice flour
- Soybean flour
- Lima bean flour

FOODS WHICH CONTAIN WHEAT

Beverages
- Beer
- Cocomalt
- Malted milk
- Postum

Breads
- Biscuit
- Crackers
- Gluten bread
- Graham bread
- Rye bread
- White bread
- Whole wheat bread
- Zwieback

Cereals
- Bran
- Cream of Wheat
- Grape Nuts
- Puffed Wheat
- Ralston
- Shredded wheat
- Wheaties

Condiments
- Mayonnaise except Miracle Whip, Ann Page, and homemade

Desserts and pastries
- Cakes and cookies
- Custards
- Doughnuts
- Dumplings
- Pie crust
- Puddings

Meats
- Hamburger meat except especially ground
- Sausages, except Armour's Brookfield and homemade

Soups
- Noodle soup
- Canned soups unless label does not list wheat

Wheat products
- Bread crumbs
- Buckwheat
- Cracker crumbs
- Macaroni
- Noodles
- Spaghetti

Miscellaneous
- Croquettes
- Gravy thickened with flour
- Griddle cakes
- Malt products
- Waffles
- Yeast cakes

Gravies may be thickened with corn starch or tapioca, or rice flour

Chicken may be fried with corn meal or without anything

Breads permitted are corn bread and Ry-Krisp

Important General Instructions Concerning Wheat-Substitute Breads

Any recipe containing wheat flour may be used by substituting:

1½ cups rolled oats, or
¾ cup potato, rice, corn, buckwheat, corn meal, or soy-bean flour, or
½ cup cornstarch
for 1 cup wheat flour

Combinations of substitutes produce better results than a single substitute; all substitutes require longer and slower baking than wheat-flour products, especially with loaf bread.

Starchy water, such as potato or rice water, makes a more moist loaf. Milk changes the flavor of the loaf, makes it richer in food value, and a more tender crumb and crust. Usually one cup of liquid is allowed for each loaf of bread the size of a loaf pan. If the dough rises too long, it will sour.

Muffins are best made in small tins so that they will be rather crusty.

If you must avoid others of the cereal grains mentioned above, such as corn, rye, etc., these cannot be used as substitutes.

FOODS WHICH CONTAIN MILK

Beverages
- Cocoa
- Chocolate
- Buttermilk
- Malted milk
- Sweet milk

Breads
- Biscuits
- Muffins
- Rolls
- White bread
- Whole wheat bread
- Corn bread

Pastries
- Cakes
- Cookies
- Custards
- Griddle cakes
- Waffles

Ice cream

Sherbets

Candies
- All chocolates

Dairy products
- Butter
- Cheese
- Condensed milk
- Cream
- Oleomargarine

Dishes prepared with milk
- Boiled salad dressing
- Creamed foods
- Escalloped dishes
- Au gratin dishes
- Gravies made with milk
- Milk or cream sauces
- Omelets with milk
- Rarebits
- Soufflés

Soups
- Bisques
- Chowders
- Milk or cream soups
- (Do not use any canned soup without reading the label)

FOODS WHICH MAY CONTAIN EGG

Beverages

- Root beer
- Malted milk
- Ovaltine

Breads

- Corn bread
- Egg bread

Breaded foods

- If the breading used is an egg mixture

Broth or consommé

- Unless known to be free of egg

Candies

- Almond cakes
- Bonbons
- Chocolates
- Fondants
- Pastes

Desserts

- Blanc mange
- Cakes
- Cookies
- Custards
- Doughnuts
- Ice cream
- Sherbets

Eggs

- Baked, coddled, deviled, fried, poached, scrambled, shirred, boiled, omelet

Pastries

- Macaroons
- Meringues
- Pies: custard, lemon, cocoanut, pumpkin
- Puddings

Salad dressings

- Mayonnaise

Sauces

- Hollandaise
- Tartar sauce

Soups

- Bouillon
- Consommé
- Mock turtle
- Noodle

Miscellaneous

- Griddle cakes
- Dumplings
- Noodles
- Pretzels
- Soufflé
- French toast
- Fritters
- Muffins
- Waffles

Meats

- Wiener schnitzel
- Meat loaf
- Croquettes

The Avoidance of Special Foods

Lists of constituents of commercial food products may be found in Vaughan and Black's *Practice of Allergy,* Rowe's *Elimination Diets,* Tuft's *Clinical Allergy,* and Morgan's *You Can't Eat That.* Furthermore, since the passage of the Food and Drug Act, nearly all prepared foods are labelled as to constituents. The patient is usually conscious of most foods which are to be avoided, but there are some whose presence may be overlooked. The more important of these are as follows:

Almond—Macaroons. Almond paste is used in many French pastries and some candies.

Apple—Apple butter. Apple pectin is used as the base of many jellies such as mint jelly. It may be present in Turkish paste candies.

Barley—Beer and ale. Scotch broth. Ovaltine. Malted milk and other malt beverages. Barley malt is used in some breakfast foods, particularly: Cornflakes, Grape-Nuts, Post Toasties, and Rice Krispies.

Beef—Many sausages. Gelatins (including Jell-O).

Buckwheat—Sometimes present in honey.

Cabbage—Sauerkraut.

Cheese—Most cheeses are made of cow's milk. Gjedoest is made from goat's milk. Roquefort (imported) is made from sheep's milk. Latticini is made from buffalo milk.

Chickory—In coffee and salads.

Chocolate—Cakes and candies. Ice creams. Medicines (often overlooked in chocolate flavored calcium tablets).

Corn—Corn Flakes. Cornmeal. Popped corn. Post Toasties, Fritos, tortillas, tamales. Hominy and hominy grits. Bourbon and corn whiskey are corn distillates and may or may not cause trouble to anyone who is allergic to corn. There are some allergists who believe that corn starch and corn sugar as well as corn oil (Mazola) are allergenic. Most of us do not agree and do not restrict these in corn-sensitive persons.

Cottonseed—It is rather generally believed now that cottonseed oil does not cause any allergic reactions and can be used without restriction. Cottonseed flour is sometimes used in bread.

Flaxseed—Roman Meal. Uncle Sam's Breakfast Food. Malt-O-Meal. Also present in flaxseed poultices, chicken feed, bird seed, wave-set, fresh paints (linseed oil).

Garlic—Some sausages. Salads.

Ginger—Gingerbread. Ginger cookies. Ginger ale. Root beer. Some spiced candies, especially the Chinese varieties.

Grapes—Dried currants. Grape juice. Raisins. Wines.

Indian Gum (Karaya Gum)—

Denture adhesive powders: Dr. Wernet's Powder, Dent-a-firm, Denture Powder, Stix.

Laxatives: many emulsified mineral oils and other laxatives, also; Bassoran (Merrell), Imbicoll (Upjohn), Karaba (Battle Creek Sanitarium), Karabim (Geo. A. Brown & Co.), Mucara (Wyeth), Saraka (Schering).

Tooth Pastes: Listerine, Lactona.

Wave sets are probably one of the most common sources.

In addition, Indian gum is found in: commercially prepared ices and flavor emulsions; certain brands of gelatin and junket; diabetic foods, including some soy bean and almond wafers; fillers for lemon, custard, and other factory made pies; fillers for ice creams and prepared ice cream powders; gum drops and candies with soft centers, as jelly beans; and hand lotions of many types.

The manufacturers of the following products state that their preparations do not contain Indian gum except as noted: Harold H. Clapp, Inc., Baby Foods; Jell-O, Jell-O Puddings, and D-Zerta, except Jell-O Ice Cream Powder; Junket Preparations except the Junket Brand Freezing Mix for ice cream; Knox Gelatin; Kremel Desserts; Royal Puddings and Royal Gelatin Desserts (standard brands).

The term "vegetable gum" on a label may mean that the preparation contains Indian gum.

Mustard—Hot sauces. Some imported sardines. Mustard plasters. Mustard pickles. Mustard seeds. Salad dressing.

Nuts—Shaved or chopped nuts or soybeans often present on rolls, cookies, and cakes.

Okra—Gumbo soups. Pepper pot soup.

Peanuts—Peanut butter. Some candies. Peanut oil is used as a base for some medicines used in injections such as Adrenalin in oil, hormones, and bismuth.

Peppers, red and green—Chili sauces. Pimento olives. Relishes. Salads.

Pork—Jell-O. Sausages. Vegetables, such as beans cooked with pork and bacon.

Soybean—Chinese soy sauce. Soybean flour. Some commercial breads. Sweet chocolate. Mull-Soy and So-Bee (milk-substitutes). Substitute for chopped nuts in biscuits, candy, etc.

Yeast—Beer. Ales. Wines. Raised breads. Medicines, such as certain vitamin preparations.

Foods Which May Be Used to Supplement a Greatly Restricted Diet

The following foods cause allergic symptoms infrequently (probably in great measure because we do not eat them much or often). Continued use might produce sensitization, but this is not extremely probable and if sensitization should occur, they are foods which can be easily avoided, thereafter. They should not be added to a prescribed diet without the knowledge of your doctor. (See list, pages 162 and 163.)

Allspice
Arrowroot
Artichoke
Avocado

Bamboo shoots
(canned Chinese)
Blackberry
Brazil nut

Cashew nut
Chestnut
Cloves
Cranberry
Currant

Dandelion wine
Date
Dewberry
Duck

Fig
Filbert
Frog legs

Gooseberry
Guava

Hazelnut

Jerusalem artichoke

Maple syrup
Maté
Molasses

Nutmeg

Okra
Olive (unstuffed)
Oyster plant

Parsley
Parsnip
Pear
Pepper (black)
Pistachio

Rhubarb

Sago
Salsify
Sesame oil

Tapioca
Terrapin
Turkey

Vinegar

Water chestnuts
(canned Chinese)

Check-Off List of Foods*

A patient may, upon receiving a long list of foods which must be avoided, exclaim with dismay "But, what *may* I eat?" The list appears so formidable that one is inclined to wonder, really, whether there is anything left to eat. However, if one has a list of those foods customarily eaten, most of which are readily available, one will find, after checking off those which must be avoided, that there is really a long list remaining.

*For a detailed discussion of the history and relationships of the various foods and for the possible ingredients of various culinary preparations, breakfast foods, nationally distributed canned, bottled or packaged foods, etc., see Vaughan and Black's *Practice of Allergy*. Your doctor can, by referring to this more technical volume, advise you concerning those preparations which may be of importance to you.

The following edible foods are arranged in accordance with their botanical classification, in such a way that one may readily recognize those which are botanically related and which might cross-react as described in Chapter VIII.

EDIBLE PLANTS

(1) SEAWEEDS

Agar-agar
Irish moss

(2) FUNGI

Mushrooms
Truffle
Puff balls
Molds
Yeast

(3) GYMNO-SPERMS

Pine nut

ANGIOSPERMS—MONOCOTYLEDONOUS FOODS

(4) CEREAL GRAINS*

Wheat **Barley** **Oat** **Wild rice**
Rye **Malt** **Rice** **Corn**

(5) **THE PALM FAMILY**

Coconut Date **Jujube**

(6) **PINEAPPLE. This fruit is not closely related to any other food.**

(7) **BANANA. This also has no closely related food, except plantain, which is not available in this country.**

(8) **THE LILY FAMILY**

Onion
Garlic
Chive
Leek
Shallot
Asparagus
Scallion

ANGIOSPERMS—DICOTYLEDONOUS FOODS

(9) **THE MULBERRY FAMILY**

Mulberry
Hop
Fig
Breadfruit

(10) **THE BUCKWHEAT FAMILY**

Rhubarb
Buckwheat

*The cereal grains and potato provide the chief source of starchy food. Occasionally nearly all of the cereal grains must be avoided. In this case the following sources of starchy foods, not closely related to other foods, may be drawn upon.

Arrowroot Cassava Tapioca
Sago (Florida Arrowroot or Indian Bread Root)

(11) THE WALNUT FAMILY
- Walnut
- Pecan
- Hickory

(12) THE BEECH FAMILY
- Chestnut
- Filbert
- Beechnut

(13) THE BEET FAMILY
- Swiss chard
- Beet
- Spinach

(14) THE GOOSEBERRY FAMILY
- Currant
- Gooseberry

(15) THE CABBAGE OR MUSTARD FAMILY
- Turnip
- Rutabaga
- Cabbage
- Kale
- Collard
- Cauliflower
- Broccoli
- Brussels sprouts
- Kohlrabi
- Mustard
- Radish
- Horse-radish
- Water cress

(16) THE ROSE FAMILY
- Strawberry
- Raspberry
- Blackberry
- Dewberry
- Loganberry

(17) THE APPLE FAMILY
- Apple*
- Apple butter
- Crab apple
- Quince
- Pear

(18) THE PLUM FAMILY
- Peach
- Nectarine
- Apricot
- Almond
- Plum
- Prune
- Cherry

(19) THE LEGUMES
- Lentil
- Kidney bean
- Lima bean
- String bean
- Blackeye pea
- Soybean
- Pea
- Peanut

(20) THE FLAX FAMILY
- Flaxseed (Linseed)

(21) THE CITROUS FAMILY
- Citron
- Orange
- Tangerine
- Bergamot
- Lemon
- Grapefruit
- Lime
- Limequat
- Kumquat

(22) THE PISTACHIO FAMILY
- Pistachio nut

*Apple pectin is widely used in commercial jellies such as mint jelly and in some candy such as Turkish paste and gum drops.

(23) THE GRAPE FAMILY
- Grape
- Raisin
- Currant (dried)
- Wine
- Brandy

(24) THE MALLOW FAMILY
- Cottonseed
- Okra (gumbo)

(25) THE CHOCOLATE FAMILY
- Chocolate
- Cocoa
- Cocoa butter

(26) THE TEA FAMILY
- Tea

(27) THE CARROT FAMILY
- Carrot
- Parsnip
- Parsley
- Celery
- Celeriac
- Fennel
- Caraway seed
- Coriander
- Anise seed
- Dill

(28) THE LAUREL FAMILY
- Cinnamon
- Avocado or alligator pear
- Bay leaves

(29) THE HUCKLEBERRY FAMILY
- Huckleberry
- Blueberry
- Cranberry

(30) THE OLIVE FAMILY
- Olive

(31) THE MORNING GLORY FAMILY
- Yam
- Sweet potato

(32) THE MINT FAMILY
- Mint
- Sage
- Savory
- Thyme

(33) THE POTATO FAMILY
- Irish potato
- Tomato
- Red and green peppers
- Eggplant

(34) THE COFFEE FAMILY
- Coffee

(35) THE GOURD FAMILY
- Squash
- Pumpkin
- Cucumber
- Watermelon
- Cantaloupe
- Muskmelon
- Honeydew

(36) THE THISTLE FAMILY
- Lettuce
- Salsify (oyster plant)
- Endive
- Chicory
- Jerusalem artichoke
- Artichoke
- Dandelion

EDIBLE ANIMAL FOODS

SEAFOODS

- Abalone
- Mussel
- Crayfish
- Shrimp

Oyster
Scallop
Clam
Squid
Lobster
Prawn
Crab
True fishes
Caviar (usually sturgeon)
Sardine

AMPHIBIANS AND REPTILES

Terrapin
Rattlesnake meat
Frog legs

BIRDS

Various types of fowl
Eggs

MAMMALIAN FOODS

Lamb
Mutton
Beef
Veal
Game
Ham
Bacon
Pork
Milk
Cream
Butter
Goat's milk
Cow's milk cheese
Goat's milk cheese
Sheep's milk cheese

The following substitute foods may be obtained from many grocers.

Starchy Foods and Wheat Flour Substitutes

Rye flour
Potato flour
Rice flour
Oat flour
Lentil flour
Green pea flour
Soy bean flour
Lima bean flour
Buckwheat (specify pure water ground)
Arrowroot
Water chestnut*
Tapioca
Sago
Hominy (corn)
Tostados (Mexican corn chips) (Fritos)
Brown rice
Wild rice
Ry-Krisp
Safemix

Fruits

Guava
Loganberry
Nectarine
Gooseberry
Kumquat
Mango
Quince
Damson plum
Green gage plum

---

*The Chinese "Water Chestnut" is a starchy tuber with chestnut flavor.

Spices and Seasonings

Cassia buds	Caraway
Cardamom	Soy sauce
Capers	Wine vinegar
Bay leaves	Cider vinegar
Anise seed	Malt vinegar

Vegetables

Bamboo shoots
Soybean sprouts
Truffles
Canned artichokes
Okra

Meats

Goose liver
Terrapin meat
Frog legs
Snails

Oils

Corn oil (Mazola)
Peanut oil
Pompeian Virgin olive oil

Beverages

Maté (tea substitute)
Postum

Nuts

Litchi nut
Pignolia (pine nut)
Almond meal

Cheese

Gjedost (goat cheese)
Imported Roquefort (sheep milk cheese)
(Specify the original imported)

Since there are various brands of many of these, some of which contain other ingredients in addition, it is well always to specify the unmixed food substances desired, with the reason therefor.

Substitute flours and other foods may be obtained from the better groceries in most cities and towns.

The following imported foods and spices are quite generally **available.**

Brazil nut (niggertoe)	Caper
Cashew nut	Clove
Guava	Allspice
Elderberry	Licorice
Nutmeg (mace)	Vanilla

Directions for Autogenous Dust Collection

There is a great deal of evidence that the active allergenic constituent of house dust is the same in various parts of the country. Sometimes, however, for some special reason it may be wise to test patients with extracts of their own dusts. We should like to do this now so we would like you to bring in samples of your own house dust. Most of the dust allergen is derived from curtains, rugs, etc., and for this reason it is important to get dust direct from furniture, mattresses, draperies and the like. The substance which causes allergic reactions in house dust is apt to be more concentrated when obtained from this source than when obtained by the ordinary manner of collection from the floor.

We therefore will want two kinds of dust. The first is the ordinary floor dust and may be obtained from the bag of the vacuum cleaner or inside of the carpet sweeper or may be brushed up from under furniture, in closets, behind pictures, etc. Collect as much as a cupful of this kind of dust, placing it in a suitable container such as a cardboard ice cream box and label it "House Dust," with your name added. Do not worry about the dust containing extraneous substances, since this will all be sterilized and only the allergenic substances will be extracted for use in testing.

Next, remove the bag from the vacuum cleaner and place on the outlet, in its stead, a clean square of old thick linen or muslin about the size of a man's handkerchief, to make a small bag, fastening it on with a rubber band or string around the outlet. Run the vacuum cleaner over the mattress and pillows, top and bottom, to get a tablespoonful of lint and dust if possible and wrap this up in the muslin. Label it, "Mattress dust," with your name added.

Next, do the same thing with any overstuffed furniture, particularly in any rooms in which you feel your symptoms are more pronounced. Keep these samples separate and label them appropriately.

If you have heavy draperies in the house, do likewise with them. If you have trouble when in your automobile, do the same with the upholstery in the car.

If you work away from home, try to get a dust specimen from your place of work.

Send these all in, properly labeled and with your name and address.

It requires from a week to ten days to complete the extraction of these substances. After that time you may report to the office for testing.

Directions for Food Diary

Occasionally a substance which actually causes trouble may fail to give a positive skin reaction. This is especially so with regard to foods. In order to detect these false negative reactors we have recourse to the food diary. It is therefore very important that the food diary be kept most accurately and that all allergic symptoms or symptoms which might be allergic be recorded in the proper place. The form we are presenting here was prepared by Drs. Rinkel and Bowen and has proved very easy to use and very helpful.

Directions for Use of the Food Diary

As you will see there are two vertical rows listing the various foods, and blank spaces are available for the writing in of additional foods. At the top of the sheet there are columns headed by letters which are for the use of the physician, then the numerals refer to the days of the month. You are expected to place a checkmark in the proper square opposite the name of the food eaten and under the proper date. This gives a record of when each food was eaten and what foods constituted the intake for each day. Since the time of day at which the food is eaten may be of importance, you will use the figure 1 to indicate breakfast, 2 for lunch, 3 for dinner and 4 if the food was used at all three meals.

At the bottom of the right-hand sheet appears the word "Symptoms." You should place opposite this and under each date your evaluation of the amount of trouble you had each day. If symptoms are entirely absent place 0 in the square. If your symptoms are slight designate them by 1; if worse, by 2 and if severe, by 3. This tells the allergist how much trouble you had each day and this can be correlated with the diet record to see whether any certain food or foods appear related to the appearance or increase of symptoms.

The line showing the word "Medicine" may be used to show the number of times each day medication is used for relief, and in the weather line you may use R for rain; N indicates a cold north wind; U shows that the weather was generally unsatisfactory and the space is left blank to indicate a good, clear day.

On the reverse of this sheet is the Allergic Time Table. This is useful in showing the time of onset of attacks and their duration. It is not of value with conditions like chronic eczema in which changes in severity are gradual and sometimes require a day or two to become evident. But in intermittent asthma, headaches, attacks of urticaria, and other conditions which show attacks with periods of freedom, this "clock" may

ALLERGIC DIET SURVEY

EGETABLES	1	2	3	4	5	6	7	8	9	10	11	12	13	14	15	16	17	18	19	20	21	22	23	24	25	26	27	28	29	3
sparagus																														
Beans, Lima																														
Beans, St.																														
Beans, Soy																														
Beets																														
Broccoli																														
B. Sprouts																														
Cabbage																														
Carrots																														
Cauliflower																														
Corn																														
Celery																														
Cucumber																														
Eggplant																														
Mustard Greens																														
Onion																														
Peas, green																														
Peas, B. E.																														
Potato, sweet																														
Potato, white																														
Radish																														
Spinach																														
Squash																														
Tomatoes																														
Turnips																														
NUTS																														
Almond																														
Brazil Nuts																														
Cashews																														
Coconut																														
Hazelnut																														
Peanut																														
Pecan																														
Pistachio																														
Walnut, black																														
Walnut, English																														
CEREALS																														
Barley																														
Buckwheat																														
Cornmeal																														
Oats																														
Rice																														
Rye																														
Wheat																														
BEVERAGES																														
Chocolate																														
Coca-Cola																														
Coffee																														
Dr. Pepper																														
Tea																														

RUITS	1	2	3	4	5	6	7	8	9	10	11	12	13	14	15	16	17	18	19	20	21	22	23	24	25	26	27	28	29	30	31
ple																															
ricot																															
nana																															
ackberry																															
ntaloupe																															
erry																															
te																															
g																															
ape																															
apefruit																															
mon																															
me																															
ive																															
ange																															
ach																															
ar																															
neapple																															
une																															
spberry																															
rawberry																															
atermelon																															
ONDIMENTS																															
nnamon																															
oves																															
nger																															
itmeg																															
prika																															
pper, black																															
mento																															
ge																															
nilla																															
EATS-DAIRY																															
ef																															
tfish																															
icken																															
ck																															
g																															
alibut																															
llo																															
mb																															
ver																															
lk																															
rk																															
lmon																															
out																															
rkey																															
na																															
MPTOMS																															

be quite helpful in giving the physician an accurate picture of the behavior of the condition.

We have found this form of record the easiest to keep with a maximum of easily interpreted information. Since there are many food sensitivities which do not show any skin reactions, this type of investigation is to be used frequently and is of great help.

Directions for Food Additions

Not all substances which give positive reactions actually cause trouble. A positive reaction indicates, rather, that that substance may be causing trouble. In our experience, on an average about one-half of the positively reacting substances actually cause trouble. However, in your individual case the proportion may be higher or lower.

Since there is no way of telling from the skin tests which of the positively reacting substances do cause trouble and which do not, the simplest procedure with which to start will be to avoid as many of the positively reacting substances as possible. As soon as adequate relief is obtained you may try exposure to some of the prohibited substances to see whether they are actual causes of trouble. With the foods for example, the diet at the beginning may be quite rigidly restricted. However after we have decided that relief has been sufficient to justify doing so, you may proceed to add one food after another to the diet, in this way determining which ones do and which do not cause trouble.

If you have been on an "elimination diet" of any kind and have lost your symptoms we would assume that you are not sensitive to any food in that diet. You may then add foods one at a time to try to detect, by its addition to the diet, which one or ones may be responsible for the symptoms.

When this is being done, it does not suffice to try the eating of a prohibited food just once and, in the absence of a return of symptoms, to conclude that that food is harmless. One can often eat an offending food occasionally and remain free from symptoms. But if it is eaten several days in succession, trouble may ensue. In the majority of cases the eating of a food on four days in succession suffices for trial. The single food to be tested is added to the diet every day for four days. If at the end of that time there has been no return of symptoms, it may be assumed that this food will not cause symptoms, and it may then be added to the regular diet. The next food should then be tried, likewise for four days in succession. Of course, if symptoms ensue in less time than the four days, the food need not be continued throughout the trial period.

In making the addition of new food one should be certain that he is adding the one food and nothing else. For example, if one adds tomato he may not eat tomato with mayonnaise on it unless egg has already been found to cause no trouble, nor should he eat cream of tomato soup unless milk has previously been found not to cause trouble. Another very important point is to see that an adequate amount of the food is eaten each day. This means that one should eat as much of the food each day as he is ever likely to eat in any one day. If you have no symptoms from this amount you may be sure you will not have trouble from this food at any later date. However, if you are testing egg and eat only one spoonful of egg each day, you may prove that one spoonful of egg does not produce symptoms but that does not mean that two eggs eaten in one day may not cause a lot of trouble.

Then, too, if the eating of a certain food brings on a recurrence of symptoms, stop the eating of that food and do not start eating another new food until the symptoms have cleared up. Otherwise, you will not be able to determine whether the new food is causing trouble or if it is only the continuation of symptoms from the preceding food.

Directions for Keeping the Inhalant Diary and the Contact Diary

The accompanying forms are applicable for the continuous study of either contact allergic dermatitis or inhalant allergy. Their use will be exemplified as applied to contact allergy.

There are two forms. Form 1 covers exposures for only one day. For convenience it is divided into three-hour periods, except during the night. The major accomplishment of such a diary will be in making the individual conscious of all contacts through the day. Let us assume that the dermatitis involves the hands. One will record on the first day all substances to which the hands are routinely exposed by contact. In the first three hours this may, for example, include comb, brush, hair tonic, toilet paper, soap, toothpaste, cigarette, matches, specified foods, newspapers, gloves, the steering wheel of an automobile, dog hair, horse hair, the nickel or bakelite handle of a dictating machine, typewriter ribbon, carbon paper, cosmetics, and the like.

Usual contacts may vary with different days of the week. Thus in the case of newspapers, one handles the colored supplement and rotogravure on Sunday but not on other days. The housewife who works in the kitchen on the servant's day off experiences different exposures at this time. The man who visits the barber shop or the woman who patronizes the beauty parlor every second week must take this into consideration. These last would be classed as unusual exposures.

INHALANT OR CONTACT DIARY (1-DAILY RECORD)

TIME	CUSTOMARY ROUTINE	UNUSUAL CONTACTS	SYMPTOM SEVERITY
6-9 A.M.			
9-12 M.			
12-3 P.M.			
3-6 P.M.			
6-9 P.M.			
9-12 MID.			
12-6 A.M.			

INHALANT OR CONTACT DIARY (2-WEEKLY RECORD)

	TIME	UNUSUAL CONTACTS AND REMARKS	SYMPTOM SEVERITY
Sunday	6-9 A.M.		
	9-12 M.		
	12-3 P.M.		
	3-6 P.M.		
	6-9 P.M.		
	9-12 MID.		
	12-6 A.M.		
Monday	6-9 A.M.		
	9-12 M.		
	12-3 P.M.		
	3-6 P.M.		
	6-9 P.M.		
	9-12 MID.		
	12-6 A.M.		
Tuesday	6-9 A.M.		
	9-12 M.		
	12-3 P.M.		
	3-6 P.M.		
	6-9 P.M.		
	9-12 MID.		
	12-6 A.M.		
Wednesday	6-9 A.M.		
	9-12 M.		
	12-3 P.M.		
	3-6 P.M.		
	6-9 P.M.		
	9-12 MID.		
	12-6 A.M.		
Thursday	6-9 A.M.		
	9-12 M.		
	12-3 P.M.		
	3-6 P.M.		
	6-9 P.M.		
	9-12 MID.		
	12-6 A.M.		
Friday	6-9 A.M.		
	9-12 M.		
	12-3 P.M.		
	3-6 P.M.		
	6-9 P.M.		
	9-12 MID.		
	12-6 A.M.		
Saturday	6-9 A.M.		
	9-12 M		
	12-3 P.M.		
	3-6 P.M.		
	6-9 P.M.		
	9-12 MID.		
	12-6 A.M.		

During the first week or two a person with contact dermatitis will spend most of his time becoming conscious of and recording his usual contact exposures. At the end of this time he will have listed them accurately for each day of the week. In the meantime he will have commenced recording unusual exposures. He will also record those days or periods of the day in which his symptom is exaggerated.

After the customary routine has been accurately recorded, it will be filed for future reference or comparison. Thereafter, only unusual contacts need be recorded. For this purpose the diary schedule 2 will be used, each sheet providing for an entire week of the record.

If the diary is being kept as an inhalant record it may well include such items for the first hours of the morning as perfume, cosmetics, dog hair, cat hair, dust from the feathers of canary birds or parrots, tooth powder, kitchen odors and gases, after-shave powders, burning wood or paper, toilet articles, gasoline exhaust fumes, change from warm air to cold air or vice versa, flowers and the like. There are usually so many contact or inhalant exposures in one's daily life that the doctor or anyone except yourself will find it practically impossible to analyze adequately the Inhalant or Contact Diary in order to find offending substances. The diary is for your own use so that you may systematize your own study and probably find things that you yourself will suspect. The doctor will then be able to do appropriate tests and see whether your suspicions are justified.

Directions to the Patient for Hypodermic Administration

Patients must sometimes give their own injections of epinephrine (Adrenalin). Occasionally they must also inject their own treatment extracts. The following instructions will be helpful.

Obtain a tuberculin syringe and a half-dozen rustless-steel hypodermic needles. These should be about ½" long and 26 gauge. The 1 c.c. tuberculin syringes are graduated in hundredths of a cubic centimeter. The larger lines, with wider spaces between them, on the Allergy Syringe, are twentieths and tenths. The figures, 20, 40, 60, etc., on the other side of the scale, mean 20/100, 40/100, etc., or two tenths, four tenths, etc. In your directions 0.01 c.c. means one one-hundredth of a cubic centimeter or the smallest graduation, and 0.1 c.c. means one-tenth of a cubic centimeter which is the distance between two of the longest white lines. You should also keep on hand some bathing alcohol and sterile cotton. The cotton in the carton as purchased does not need further sterilization.

Insert the plunger into the barrel of the syringe after discarding the small piece of cork. Remove the wire from the needle and discard the wire. Place the needle securely on the tip of syringe with a slight twisting motion. Wrap in a small piece of gauze or other clean cloth and place in a saucepan containing about 1 inch of water. Boil for ten minutes. The syringe is now sterile, so when you remove it from the pan be careful not to touch the needle or allow it to come in contact with anything (except that you should grasp the needle by the hub and twist it slightly to be sure that it is tight on the syringe).

Wet a small piece of cotton with rubbing alcohol and wipe off the rubber cap on the bottle of extract. Do not remove this cap. Pull the plunger back to the same point on the syringe that you are going to use for your dosage. Insert the needle through the center of the rubber cap. Push the plunger all the way in, to expel the air into the bottle. Invert the bottle and carefully withdraw into the syringe 1 c.c. (100 hundredths) of the extract. Then, with the needle still pointing up push the plunger in to the desired dosage mark on the barrel of the syringe. This will expel all of the air bubbles in the syringe. If it does not do so, refill the syringe and again push the plunger back to the desired point. Gently tapping the syringe with the tip of the finger will help dislodge air bubbles.

Withdraw the needle from the bottle, taking care not to disturb the position of the plunger and being careful not to contaminate the needle. Use the outer part of the upper arm or inner portion of the thigh (do not use the inner part of the upper arm). Sponge a small area of the skin with the piece of cotton used to wipe off the cap of the vial. If the arm is used, bend the elbow to make the skin taut. Hold the syringe between the first and second fingers with the thumb pressing gently against the side of the plunger. Quickly plunge the needle through the sterilized area of the skin at an angle of 45 degrees. It should be inserted rapidly and to the hub of the needle. This makes the injection practically painless. The thumb then is moved to the end of the plunger and gently pressed all the way in. When removing the needle, do it quickly, since this minimizes the discomfort. If the thigh is used, the left hand is used to stretch the skin. Withdraw the needle and wipe the area again with the alcohol sponge. It is a good precaution, after inserting the needle and before pressing down on the plunger, to exert gentle suction with the plunger to be sure that no blood comes back into the syringe. If it does, the needle may be in a small vein and the needle should be withdrawn and reinserted at another point ½ inch away. This suction can be applied, while still holding the syringe, with the little finger wrapped around the end of the plunger.

Always keep the needle sharp, as a needle with a dull or bent point will hurt much more than a sharp one. The needle may be sharpened with a fine carborundum stone. However, do not hesitate to use a new needle.

If you do not wish to be bothered with sterilizing the syringe each time, you may obtain a special pocket apparatus* containing a harmless liquid antiseptic.†

Your extract contains______________________________________.

You should take the injections every ______ day and the dose of each injection is:

1st	____________c.c.	6th	____________c.c.
2nd	____________c.c.	7th	____________c.c.
3rd	____________c.c.	8th	____________c.c.
4th	____________c.c.	9th	____________c.c.
5th	____________c.c.	10th	____________c.c.

Check off each succeeding injection as you take it so that you will neither repeat nor skip a dose in the sequence.

When you have completed this course of treatment, please communicate with us.

A Medical Life-Record

The study of disease is the study of the processes of living. Human disease terminates at death. Allergy, the process of reacting in an altered manner, cannot continue when there is no longer something which can react. On the other hand, living persons are capable of responding abnormally to environmental stimuli from birth, even from conception, and until the last moment of life.

If we are to learn more about allergy, it becomes important to study the disease in its incipiency, in its earliest manifestations, and to follow the alterations in these manifestations, onward through the life of the individual. As more knowledge is gained in this way, we shall reach a clearer understanding and, as a consequence, evolve better methods for prevention and treatment.

*"Steritube" (Becton, Dickenson & Co.)

†Bard-Parker sterilizing fluid.

A permanent written record of the medical life-history of every child, particularly of every child born into an allergic family, might well be started at birth. The old family Bible may contain a record of one's birth and facilitate tracing of one's ancestry, but of far greater interest to the individual should be his own subsequent experiences and those of others yet to come, who will look back to him as an ancestor. The past has passed, but the future holds the possibility of human control and alteration, within certain limits. The allergic patient of this generation can aid his allergic children of the next, by helping doctors to reach a clearer insight into the life-history of the disease.

It has been a delightful custom to give proud parents a pretty little book bound in pink or blue, entitled "Baby's Life." In it one finds charmingly decorated pages, with many spaces for photographs, and with provision for a record of "Baby's first smile . . . baby's first word . . . . baby's first tooth . . . . baby walked. . . ." Usually there is some genealogical record with provision for the names of parents and grandparents, aunts and uncles. Some of the more advanced books provide for records of the dates of the usual diseases of childhood and some even give space for records of smallpox vaccination, Schick tests, and diphtheria prophylaxis.

How much more valuable these books would become to the allergic individual if they were designed to contain records of the potential inheritance of certain disease tendencies, so that proper steps might be taken to prevent them; record of childhood idiosyncrasies and earliest allergic manifestations, so that the tendency could be controlled before it becomes firmly established; notations of vaccinations, serum inoculations, and extract treatments with a record of how the subject responded or reacted to them, so that physicians who might see him at a later time will know the manner of his response and will be better able to give the most successful treatment.

Such a volume would be an invaluable medical dossier in which both the doctor and patient would make brief summary notations, on the patient's birthday. He would take his life-record with him when consulting a new physician to aid both the doctor and himself, and to prevent repetition of possible previous therapeutic failures.

Such records would be of greatest value to the individual. Some of them, when analyzed by competent investigators, would aid us in reaching the goal of clearer understanding of allergy.

This is an ideal which may not be easily put into execution. A publisher might produce the ideal Life-Record volume. Many might purchase it. Not so many users will, however, be sufficiently interested or persistent to keep it properly up to date at all times. Memory is indeed fallacious and inaccurately recalled notations are of less value than none at all.

There is one thing that can be done, in every instance. When the victim of allergy has placed himself under the supervision and guidance of a physician skilled in this field of medicine, it becomes the duty of the latter to inaugurate a comprehensive record, to which additions are made from time to time, particularly in the annual check-ups; a record, the contents of which may always be available to the patient. In no other field of medicine is the need for permanent detailed records more apparent. The patient who cooperates toward this end will be aiding not only himself but other sufferers from his disease.

Questions and Answers

Q. I have heard that many allergists consider inhalants much more important than foods. What is the relative importance?

A. The answer to this question probably will not be the same from any two allergists. There are some who believe that foods seldom cause allergic reactions and there are others who are sure that foods constitute the major problem in allergy. Why there should be this marked difference we are not sure. Some of it may be due to the fact that pollens which cause trouble may be few in a particular area or, on the other hand, they may be so many and so abundant that they overshadow everything else. Molds may play a very important role in certain parts of the country and be of little importance in others. Most of us believe that both inhalants and foods are important as causes of sensitivity and that results of treatment will be poor unless both are given adequate consideration. There are many patients who are definitely allergic to both inhalants and foods and in whom good results are not apparent unless both are cared for.

Q. Is sick headache always due to food allergy?

A. Not at all. Migraine is a disease, the acute episodes of which may be brought on by quite a large number of exciting causes. In a predisposed person this kind of headache may be brought on by nonallergic factors such as constipation, an abscessed tooth, fatigue, emotional upsets, eyestrain or by allergic factors, especially by foods. In my experience allergenic foods are an important factor. This is probably due in part to the fact that we see so many allergic patients. Doctors working in other fields of medicine would be likely to see more migraine due to other causes and less due to food allergy. In at least 30 per cent of those patients with migrainous type of headache whom we see, we find no evidence of allergy at all.

Q. If allergic patients are usually sensitized to several things, and if you don't discover all the things a person is allergic to, how can you relieve him?

A. In the early days of allergic treatment many people were adequately relieved after just a dozen or so tests had shown them to be sensitized to one or two or three things. The probability is that if they had been tested with a hundred things many other allergens would have been positive. Nevertheless they were relieved. There is evidence indicating that if part of the allergenic overload is removed the patient will tolerate his remaining contacts or exposures more successfully (see illustrations on pages 89, 91 and 93).

This is not always true. An asthmatic woman had been treated by a leading allergist for two years without relief. When she came to us we did the same tests, found the same reactions, and would have put her on the same program except that we tested her to moth scales (a constituent of house dust) to which the other doctor had not tested her. She gave a strongly positive reaction. After that, the same treatment that the other doctor had given her *plus* desensitizing injections of moth scale extract relieved her. This case illustrates the desirability of finding all of the offenders if they can be found.

Q. My asthma is caused by ragweed. Why is it that with preventive treatment I am relieved while staying in my own home town but have trouble invariably when I go to another city which is twenty miles away, although there are no mountains, rivers, or swamps between and the agriculture and industries are the same in both places? I get worse even when driving into the city, without even going into stores, homes, gardens, etc.

A. The following case illustrates one possible answer. A boy living in Laurinburg, N. C., has had precisely that experience. He can go fifteen miles out of town in any direction and be relieved. Driving back, his asthma returns as soon as he gets inside this circle. Laurinburg is situated in a shallow, saucer-shaped basin edged by a sand ridge. Dust and pollen grains seem to settle in the basin and become concentrated there. During the tobacco and cotton season when there is much dust, a person driving at night seems to be going through a haze. As soon as one drives up over the edge of the ridge, the air becomes clear. The average person is not even conscious of the shallow basin.

We see this same situation in the coal fields of West Virginia where a pall of dust and smoke settles down in the valleys.

In other words, there are places even within a few miles of each other where allergic persons, especially those with respiratory allergy, will do well or poorly. The asthmatic in West Virginia might do better if he were just to move up near the top of the mountain, not a quarter of a mile away.

Q. My doctor has always told me that my trouble was sinus disease and now you say it is nasal allergy. How can I know which is correct?

A. One may have both nasal allergy and sinus infection. When they occur together, the latter is usually a result of a more long-standing nasal allergy. Often, however, uncomplicated nasal allergy is erroneously mistaken for sinus trouble. The same is true of recurrent head colds. A person who says, "I catch cold all the time" or "I hardly get over one cold before I get another," is likely to be suffering from nasal allergy.

There is no absolute way in which the patient himself can distinguish between the two conditions. In nasal allergy the secretion is more likely to be thin and watery while in sinus disease it is more apt to be rather thickish, whitish or yellowish, looking more like pus. With ordinary head colds, the secretion which at first is thin and watery later becomes thick, yellowish. In uncomplicated nasal allergy or hay fever it stays thin throughout the attack.

Diagnosis is especially difficult when both conditions exist. There is a laboratory test, the examination of the nasal secretion for a special kind of leukocyte, the *eosinophil,* which usually enables the doctor to tell whether allergy is playing a part.

Q. When one has a combination of nasal allergy and sinus infection, which should be treated?

A. Sometimes it is necessary to treat both, with allergen avoidance, desensitizing injections, and possibly also diet for the allergy and local treatment by a nose and throat man for the sinus infection. Our experience has been that it is best to treat the allergy first, after which the sinus infection may take care of itself. Sometimes, however, allergic treatment alone is not sufficient. If symptoms persist after allergic therapy has been given an adequate trial, local nasal treatment is given in conjunction with continued allergic treatment.

Q. I invariably sneeze half a dozen times when I get up in the morning and an electric fan is likely to produce hay fever or asthma. I get into trouble when I drive in an open automobile. Even walking along the street in the wind may cause my asthma or hay fever to return. Just about the worst thing I can do to myself is to sleep under an electric fan. Ice cream and even ice water make my nose stop up and cause coughing spells which may develop into asthma. Going from a hot place into a cold one, such as an air-conditioned building, and sometimes the reverse will make me sneeze or wheeze.

A. These are common complaints among persons with respiratory allergy. Some complain of one or several of these reactions while occasionally one complains of all.

There is a delicate adjustment of the heat-regulating mechanism in the body that keeps our temperatures always the same. If we get out in the cold or in a draft the blood vessels in the skin close down, driving the blood inward, into the internal structures including the mucous membranes of the nose. The latter become engorged or swollen as a result, and symptoms ensue. The same is true in the bronchi. When you jump out of bed and remove your night clothes, the skin responds in the same way and with similar results. This is a normal reflex but, when it occurs in a nonallergic person, he is not aware of it. It is so exaggerated in the allergic person that it may produce marked reactions. One may prevent many attacks by avoiding such sudden changes in temperature. It is an interesting fact that, if the allergic condition is controlled, these reactions to changes in temperature disappear.

Q. What can an expectant mother do to prevent her child from becoming allergic?

A. One competent allergist has produced evidence which rather strongly suggests that when an allergic pregnant woman eats excessive quantities of some food such as chocolate or nuts, a craving that sometimes does exist, the child is rather likely to become sensitized to that food as a result of the overexposure, through the mother's circulation.

The expectant mother should eat a well-balanced diet with no unnatural excesses. This should be continued through the time that the child is nursing at the breast because it has been definitely proved that food allergens eaten by the mother can be carried over in breast milk and thus delivered to the potentially allergic child.

During the last quarter century there has been a tendency on the part of child specialists to introduce new foods such as egg, toast, and cereals at a much earlier age than formerly. The mucous membrane of the infant's digestive tract is less thoroughly protected against passage of foreign protein than after it has grown older and there is thus a definite risk of producing sensitization by too early introduction of new foods. Within the last few years pediatrists have recognized this fact and more of them now postpone new foods to a somewhat later date. Nowadays, egg yolk which is less highly allergenic than egg white is introduced before whole egg is given.

Q. Do children have a natural tendency to outgrow allergy?

A. This does occur in some cases. Most cases of infantile eczema clear up around age 2 or 3. Unfortunately they are then rather likely to develop asthma instead. Boys are a little more apt to develop asthma in childhood while girls are more likely to have it after adolescence. A boy with childhood asthma sometimes clears up around adolescence.

Unfortunately one cannot count on these cures of asthma because they happen rather infrequently. In our experience we believe the percentage of those getting spontaneous cure is not greater than ten or fifteen per cent. The simplest procedure is to give adequate treatment so that if spontaneous cure does not occur, the child's symptoms will be properly controlled. Furthermore there is some evidence suggesting that proper treatment will increase the tendency to spontaneous cure.

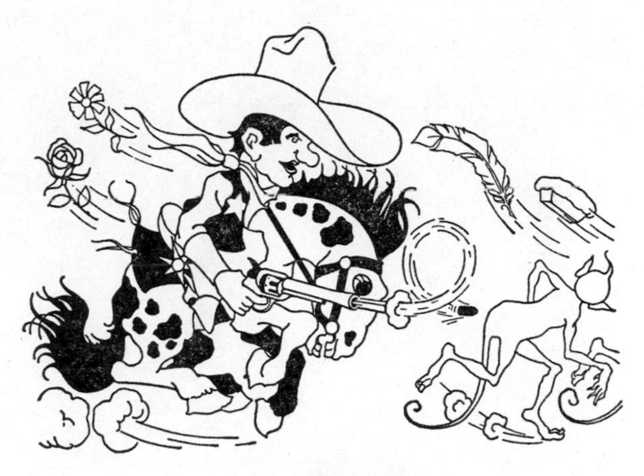

Farewell to Allergy

INDEX

S

T